Instructor's Manual

SECOND EDITION

EXERCISE PHYSIOLOGY

Theory and Application to Fitness and Performance

SCOTT K. POWERS
University of Florida

EDWARD T. HOWLEY
University of Tennessee–Knoxville

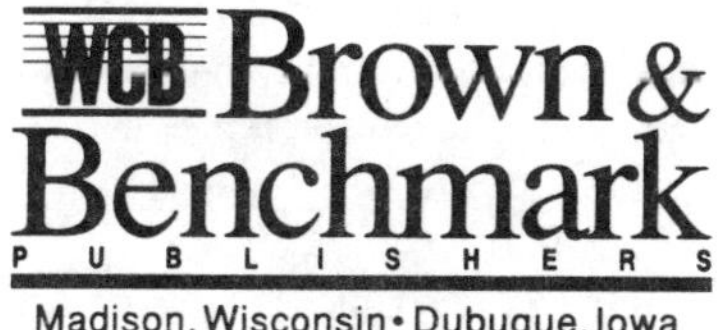

A Times Mirror Company

ISBN 0-697-12658-7

Printed in the United States of America by Wm. C. Brown Communications, Inc., 2460 Kerper Boulevard, Dubuque, Iowa, 52001

10 9 8 7 6 5 4 3 2 1

Contents

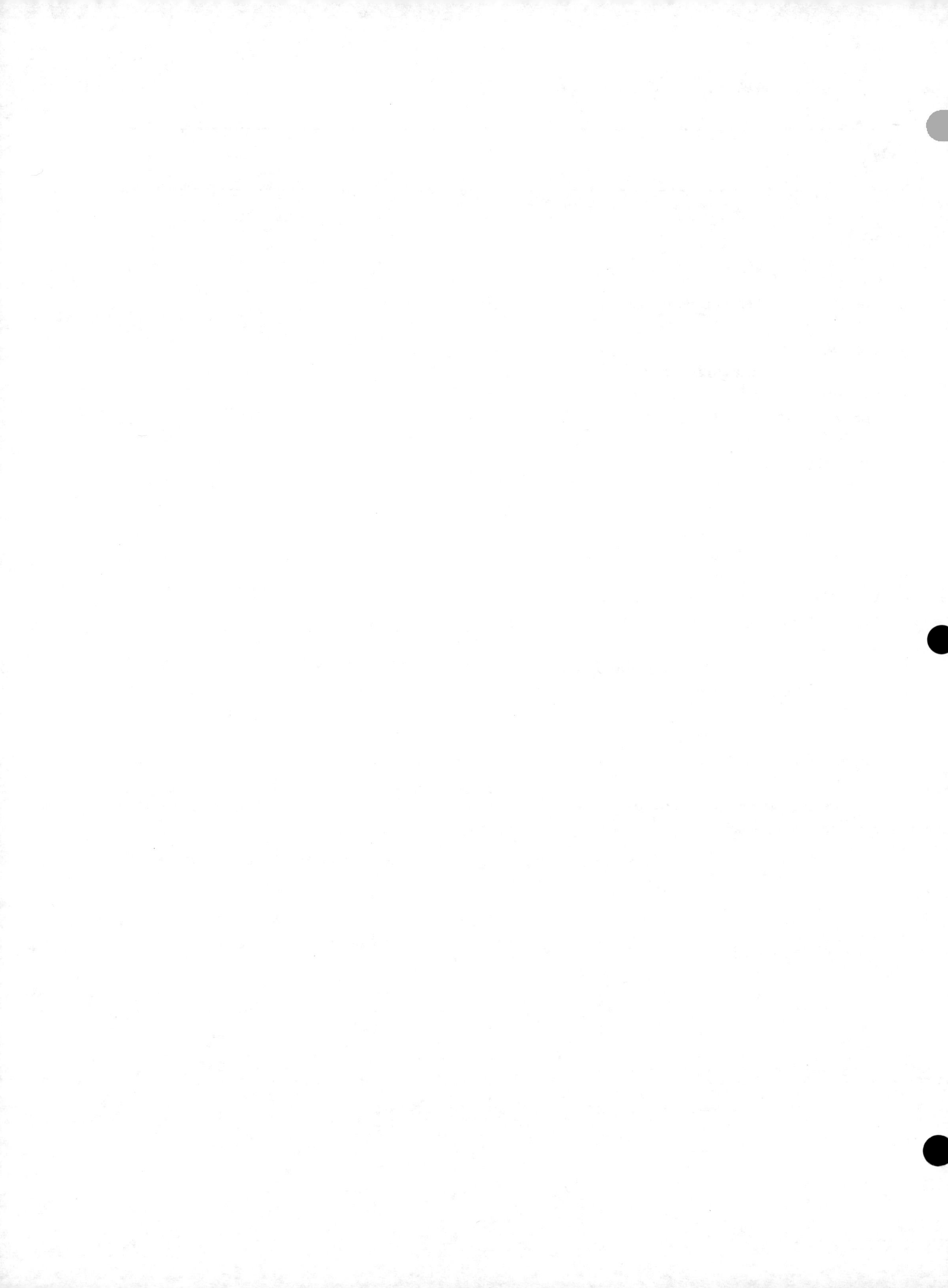

Preface

This instructor's manual is designed to assist the instructor of exercise physiology in preparation of lecture materials, exams, and laboratory experiences. This manual contains a lecture outline of each chapter of the text *Exercise Physiology: Theory and Application to Fitness and Performance.* In addition, a test bank is included as well as a list of suggested laboratory experiences. The lecture outline follows the sequence of topical presentation in the text. This outline provides a list of key points, and each key point is expanded by a list of subpoints. Many of the subpoints are illustrated via examples or additional details that might be useful to the beginning student of exercise physiology.

The test bank contains multiple choice and true/false questions that are intended for use with the undergraduate student. Correct answers follow each question. The answer to each question in the test bank can be found within the respective chapter in the text, and most questions are covered in the learning objectives of each chapter.

Finally, a list of suggested laboratory experiences is provided to assist the instructor in illustrating specific concepts in exercise physiology. These lab experiences are designed to provide the instructor with ideas for practical laboratory experiences to aid the student in learning specific concepts in exercise physiology.

Chapter 1 Physiology of Exercise in the United States—Its Past, Its Future

Lecture Outline

Key Points	*Subpoints*	*Examples*
Historical figures in physiology of exercise	Names of leaders	A. V. Hill A. Krogh O. Meyerhof J. S. Haldane C. G. Douglas
D. B. Dill and the Harvard Fatigue Laboratory	1. Work of lab 2. Foreign visitors	List types of studies done Name of prominent scientists: E. Asmussen; M. Nielsen; E. H. Christensen; R. Margaria
History of fitness in the United States	1. Past history	Dudley Sargent at Harvard
	2. Influence of war	Failing induction exam
	3. Korean Conflict	Advanced atherosclerosis in young soldiers
	4. Kraus-Weber test	U.S. children not as fit as European children
	5. President's Council on Youth Fitness	D. D. Eisenhower J. F. Kennedy
	6. Health-related fitness	AAHPERD test: cardiovascular fitness; low back function; body fatness

Key Points	*Subpoints*	*Examples*
Graduate study and research in exercise physiology	1. History	Old Harvard program
	2. Growth of university programs	Illinois (T. K. Cureton) Penn State (E. R. Buskirk) Wisconsin (B. Balke/F. Nagle)
	3. Research journals	Show examples, e.g., *Journal of Applied Physiology; Medicine and Science in Sports and Exercise*
	4. Professional societies	List examples; discuss those in which you hold membership

Exam Questions

1. The director of the Harvard Fatigue Laboratory was
   a. A. V. Hill.
   b. August Krogh.
   c. Otto Meyerhof.
   d. D. B. Dill.
   d

2. The professional society that has published a health-related fitness manual for public schools is the
   a. American College of Sports Medicine.
   b. American Alliance for Health, Physical Education, Recreation, and Dance.
   c. American Physiological Society.
   d. Association for Fitness in Business.
   b

3. Name two journals that publish research articles dealing with exercise or environmental physiology: ______________________________ and ______________________________.
   Medicine and Science in Sports and Exercise; Journal of Applied Physiology; Journal of Aviation, Space, and Environmental Medicine; etc.

Chapter 2 Control of the Internal Environment

Lecture Outline

Key Points	*Subpoints*	*Examples*
Homeostasis is defined as a constant or unchanging internal environment	Homeostasis vs. steady-state	Body temperature regulation
Control systems of the body	Goal of control systems is to regulate some physiological variable near a constant value	
Nature of control systems	1. Biological control system is a series of interconnected components serving to maintain a parameter of the body constant	Temperature regulation
	2. Components of a biological control system include a receptor, integrating center, and effector	Pressure receptors (baroreceptors), CV control center, blood vessels
	3. Most biological control systems operate via negative feedback	Respiratory control
	4. Gain of a control system is defined as amount of correction needed/amount of abnormality that exists after correction	Temperature regulation
Examples of homeostatic control		Regulation of arterial blood pressure Regulation of blood glucose

Key Points	*Subpoints*	*Examples*
Exercise is a dramatic test of homeostatic control	Severe exercise may disrupt many homeostatic variables	Muscular production of lactic acid

Exam Questions

1. The term *homeostasis* is defined as
   a. a constant metabolic demand placed upon the body.
   b. the maintenance of a constant or unchanging internal environment (i.e., usually applied to denote normal conditions during rest).
   c. a low metabolic rate.
   d. a change within the internal environment.
   b

2. Physiologists use the term *steady state* to denote
   a. a steady and unchanging internal environment.
   b. a completely normal external environment.
   c. a changing internal environment.
   d. an increase in body heat storage.
   a

3. A biological control system can be defined as
   a. a reflex arc resulting in a dynamic change in limb position.
   b. a rigid series of resistors that act to prevent an increase in blood pressure.
   c. a series of interconnected components that serve to maintain a physical or chemical parameter of the body constant.
   d. an integrating center that acts as a control box.
   c

4. The general components of a biological control system are the
   a. receptor, integrating center, and control center.
   b. receptor, integrating center, and the effector.
   c. effector, control box, and stimulus.
   d. stimulus, receptor, and integrating center.
   b

5. Most control systems of the body operate via
   a. positive feedback.
   b. low-gain receptors.
   c. negative feedback.
   d. both low-gain receptors and positive feedback.
   c

6. The gain of a biological control system can be thought of as the
   a. amount of amplification of the system or the precision with which the control system maintains homeostasis.
   b. ratio of the amount of abnormality to the amount of correction needed to maintain a constant internal environment (i.e., amount of abnormality/amount of correction needed).
   c. amount of positive feedback needed to maintain homeostasis.
   d. All of the above are correct.
   a

7. In negative feedback, the response of the control system is
   a. to increase the gain of the receptor.
   b. to modify the receptor's response to the stimulus.
   c. opposite that of the stimulus.
   d. All of the above are correct.

   c

Suggested Lab Experiences

Several laboratory experiences could be employed to improve students' understanding of biological control systems. Suggested lab experiences include:

1. *Glucose tolerance test.* The objective is to demonstrate the regulation of the blood glucose concentration following a glucose challenge. Measurements could include changes in the blood glucose concentration at selected time intervals following ingestion of a sugar solution.
2. *Respiratory response to CO_2 inhalation.* The objective is to illustrate the response of the respiratory control center to an increase in arterial CO_2. Medical grade CO_2 could be delivered to the subject from a storage tank via a mixing chamber at a fixed rate (i.e., 0.5–1.5 liters/min) and ventilation and end-tidal CO_2 tension measured.

Chapter 3 Bioenergetics

Lecture Outline

Key Points	*Subpoints*	*Examples*
Cell structure	Cell structure can be divided into three main parts: (a) cell membrane; (b) nucleus; and (c) cytoplasm	Liver cell
Biological energy transformation	First and second laws of thermodynamics: (a) Law of conservation of energy (i.e., energy cannot be created nor destroyed); (b) Energy transformations in living systems result in entropy	
Cellular chemical reactions	1. Coupled reactions 2. Role of enzymes	Lactate dehydrogenase
Fuels for exercise	1. Carbohydrates 2. Fats 3. Proteins	Glucose/glycogen FFA Amino acids
High-energy phosphates	1. Energy stored in chemical bond joining ADP & P_i 2. Structure of ATP: (a) Adenine portion; (b) Ribose portion; and (c) Three inorganic phosphates 3. ATPase catalyzes the hydrolysis of ATP and energy release	

Key Points	*Subpoints*	*Examples*
Bioenergetics	1. Anaerobic ATP production: (a) ATP-CP; (b) Glycolysis 2. Aerobic ATP production: (a) Krebs cycle (b) Electron transport chain	
Aerobic ATP tally	1. Glycolysis alone: glucose (2 ATP), glycogen (3 ATP) 2. Aerobic ATP production: glucose (38 ATP), glycogen (39 ATP)	
Regulation of bioenergetics	1. Control of ATP-CP system is accomplished via ADP/ATP stimulation or inhibition of creatine kinase activity 2. Control of glycolysis is accomplished via ADP/ATP stimulation or inhibition of PFK activity 3. Control of Krebs cycle is accomplished by regulation of isocitrate dehydrogenase activity (i.e., ADP stimulates while ATP inhibits) 4. Electron transport chain activity is regulated via the amount of ATP and ADP present	Accumulation of ADP at onset of exercise
Interaction between aerobic and anaerobic ATP production	Energy to perform most activities comes from both aerobic and anaerobic sources	400-meter run (i.e., 75% anaerobic/25% aerobic)

Exam Questions

1. The two most important functions of the cell membrane are to
   a. regulate protein synthesis and passage of materials in and out of the cell.
   b. enclose the components of the cell and to regulate passage of materials in and out of the cell.
   c. guard against cellular pH changes.
   d. enclose the components of the cell and to regulate protein synthesis.

   b

2. The organelle that regulates protein synthesis is the
   a. mitochondria.
   b. golgi apparatus.
   c. nucleus.
   d. sarcoplasmic reticulum.

   c

3. The first law of thermodynamics states that
   a. energy cannot be created nor destroyed.
   b. energy cannot be stored.
   c. energy cannot be converted into other forms.
   d. energy transformations result in an increase in entropy.

   a

4. By definition, an endergonic reaction is
   a. a chemical reaction that requires energy to be added to the reactants before the reaction will take place.
   b. a chemical reaction that gives off energy.
   c. an enzyme catalyzed reaction.
   d. None of the above are correct.

   a

5. Coupled reactions are defined as
   a. reactions that are linked together via the same enzyme.
   b. reactions that are linked together, with the liberation of free energy in one reaction being used to drive the second reaction.
   c. reactions that are not directly linked together but are related to the same enzyme.
   d. reactions that are linked via common substrates.

   b

6. Enzymes are catalysts that increase the rate of reactions by
   a. pulling two substrates together.
   b. lowering the energy of activation.
   c. binding to a substrate and producing energy.
   d. binding to a substrate and releasing protons.

   b

7. Stored polysaccharides in muscle and other tissues in animals is called
   a. glucose.
   b. fructose.
   c. glycogen.
   d. cellulose.

   c

8. Neutral fats that are stored in muscle and other tissues and play an important role as an energy substrate are
   a. phospholipids.
   b. cholesterol.
   c. triglycerides.
   d. lipoproteins.

   c

9. The most important high-energy phosphate compound in the muscle cell is
   a. NAD.
   b. FAD.
   c. ATP.
   d. GTP.

   c

10. The simplest and most rapid method to produce ATP during exercise is through
    a. glycolysis.
    b. ATP-CP system.
    c. aerobic metabolism.
    d. glycogenolysis.

    b

11. The principal function of glycolysis is to
    a. degrade glucose or glycogen into pyruvic acid or lactic acid and produce ATP.
    b. form NADH and FADH.
    c. degrade lactic acid to pyruvic acid.
    d. generate high-energy compounds such as GTP.

    a

12. The net production of ATP via substrate-level phosphorylation is glycolysis is
    a. 2 ATP if glucose is the substrate and 4 ATP if glycogen is the substrate.
    b. 2 ATP if glucose is the substrate and 3 ATP if glycogen is the substrate.
    c. 3 ATP if glucose is the substrate and 4 ATP if glycogen is the substrate.
    d. 3 ATP if glucose is the substrate and 3 ATP if glycogen is the substrate.

    b

13. The two most important hydrogen (electron) carriers in bioenergetic chemical reactions are
    a. NAD and ATP.
    b. FAD and ATP.
    c. NAD and FAD.
    d. NAD and LDH.

    c

14. The primary function of the Krebs cycle is
    a. to complete the oxidation of carbohydrates, fats, and proteins (i.e., form NADH and FADH).
    b. to produce ATP via substrate-level phosphorylation.
    c. to prime glycolysis for the production of ATP.
    d. to produce H_2O and ATP.

    a

15. Aerobic production of ATP occurs
    a. in the mitochondria in a process called glycolysis.
    b. in the mitochondria (i.e., electron transport chain) in a process called oxidative phosphorylation.
    c. in the mitochondria in a process called beta oxidation.
    d. in the cytoplasm.

    b

16. Pairs of electrons carried by NADH contain enough energy to rephosphorylate
    a. 2 ADP to form 2 ATP.
    b. 3 ADP to form 3 ATP.
    c. 4 ADP to form 4 ATP.
    d. None of the above are correct.

    b

17. The total ATP production via aerobic breakdown of glucose is
    a. 30 ATP.
    b. 36 ATP.
    c. 38 ATP.
    d. 39 ATP.

    c

18. The calculated efficiency for aerobic respiration is approximately
    a. 20%.
    b. 30%.
    c. 40%.
    d. None of the above are correct.

    c

19. The breakdown of creatine phosphate is regulated by
    a. the amount of lactate dehydrogenase in the muscle.
    b. the amount of NAD in the sarcoplasm of the muscle.
    c. ADP concentration in the cytoplasm.
    d. the pH of the interstitial fluid.

    c

20. The most important rate limiting enzyme in glycolysis is
    a. lactate dehydrogenase.
    b. hexokinase.
    c. phosphofructokinase.
    d. pyruvate kinase.

    c

21. The rate limiting enzyme in the Krebs cycle is
    a. isocitrate dehydrogenase.
    b. hexokinase.
    c. succinate dehydrogenase.
    d. None of the above are correct.

    a

22. In general, the higher the intensity of the activity, the greater the contribution of
    a. aerobic energy production.
    b. anaerobic energy production.
    c. the Krebs cycle to the production of ATP.
    d. the electron transport chain to the production of ATP.

    b

Suggested Lab Experiences

Several laboratory experiences could be employed to improve the students' understanding of bioenergetics. Suggested lab experiences include:

1. *Influence of pH and temperature on enzyme activity.* The objective is to demonstrate the influence of changes in temperature and pH on enzyme activity. Measurements on the rate of substrate formation (in vitro) under various pH and temperature conditions could be performed on any number of commercially available biological enzymes.
2. *Blood lactic acid alterations during exercise.* The objective is to demonstrate the change in blood lactic acid concentrations following various activities (i.e., 50-meter dash, 100-meter dash, 400-meter dash, 5000 meter run etc.)

Chapter 4 Exercise Metabolism

Lecture Outline

Key Points	*Subpoints*	*Examples*
Metabolic responses to exercise	1. Rest to work transitions—O_2 deficit	Start of exercise
	2. Short-term intense exercise	100-meter dash
	3. Prolonged exercise	10-K run
	4. Incremental exercise	Stress test
	5. Lactate threshold—controversy exists as to cause—may be due to cellular hypoxia, fiber recruitment patterns, rising blood levels of catecholamines, and/or alterations in the rate of lactate removal from blood	
	6. Practical use of lactate threshold	Prediction of performance
Estimation of fuel utilization during exercise	R.Q. useful during steady-state work in estimating substrate utilization during exercise	R.Q. = 1.0 = 100% CHO R.Q. = .07 = 100% Fat R.Q. = 0.85 = 50% CHO 50% Fat

Key Points	*Subpoints*	*Examples*
Factors governing fuel selection	1. Regulation of protein metabolism—dependent upon CHO stores and availability of branched chained amino acids 2. Regulation of carbohydrate metabolism—dependent upon CHO stores and phosphorylase activity 3. Regulation of fat metabolism—dependent upon intensity and duration of activity—rate of lipolysis controlled by lipase activity 4. Interaction of fat and carbohydrate metabolism—CHO necessary for fat metabolism	
Recovery from exercise: metabolic responses	Oxygen debt due to: (a) Rapid portion—restoration of O_2 stores in blood and tissues and resynthesis of CP; (b) Slow portion—Q_{10} effect	

Exam Questions

1. The first bioenergetic pathway to become active at the onset of exercise is
   a. glycolysis.
   b. the ATP-CP system.
   c. the Krebs cycle.
   d. the electron transport chain.
   b

2. The term *oxygen deficit* refers to the
   a. lag in oxygen consumption at the beginning of exercise.
   b. excess oxygen consumption during recovery from exercise.
   c. amount of oxygen required to maintain a steady state during constant load exercise.
   d. None of the above are correct.
   a

3. Energy to run a maximal 400-meter race (i.e., 50 to 60 seconds) comes from
   a. aerobic metabolism exclusively.
   b. mostly aerobic metabolism with some anaerobic metabolism.
   c. a combination of aerobic/anaerobic metabolism with most of the ATP coming from anaerobic sources.
   d. the ATP-CP system exclusively.

   c

4. Energy to run a 40-yard dash comes
   a. almost exclusively from the ATP-CP system.
   b. exclusively from glycolysis.
   c. almost exclusively from aerobic metabolism.
   d. from a combination of aerobic/anaerobic metabolism, with most of the ATP being produced aerobically.

   a

5. The energy to perform long-term exercise (i.e., > 15 min) comes primarily from
   a. aerobic metabolism.
   b. a combination of aerobic/anaerobic metabolism, with anaerobic metabolism producing the bulk of the ATP.
   c. anaerobic metabolism.
   d. None of the above are correct.

   a

6. The lactate threshold is defined as
   a. the work rate or oxygen uptake where there is a systematic rise in blood levels of lactic acid.
   b. the work rate or oxygen uptake where there is a systematic rise in aerobic metabolism.
   c. the work rate or oxygen uptake where there is a systematic decrease in blood lactic acid concentration.
   d. All of the above are correct.

   a

7. The lactate threshold is possibly due to
   a. a lack of oxygen in the muscle cell.
   b. recruitment of fast-twitch fibers and a form of LDH that favors lactate production.
   c. a reduced rate of removal of lactic acid from the blood.
   d. All of above are correct.
   e. None of above are correct.

   d

8. A respiratory quotient (RQ) of 0.95 during steady-state exercise is suggestive of a(n)
   a. high rate of carbohydrate metabolism.
   b. high rate of fat metabolism.
   c. equal rate of fat/carbohydrate metabolism.
   d. high rate of protein metabolism.

   a

9. The contribution of protein to the fuel supply toward the completion of two hours of aerobic exercise in a normal state of nutrition may reach
   a. 1%–2%.
   b. 2%–4%.
   c. 5%–15%.
   d. 20%–30%.

   c

10. Most of the carbohydrate (e.g., for a rested, well-fed athlete) used as a substrate during exercise comes from
    a. muscle glycogen stores.
    b. blood glucose.
    c. liver glycogen stores.
    d. glycogen stored in fat cells.

    a

11. The process of breaking down triglycerides into free fatty acids and glycerol is called
    a. beta oxidation.
    b. glycogenolysis.
    c. lipolysis.
    d. Both (a) and (c) are correct.

    c

12. Depletion of carbohydrate stores during exercise influences fat metabolism by
    a. increasing the amount of muscle lactic acid production.
    b. reducing the amount of pyruvic acid in the sarcoplasm, resulting in a conversion of oxaloacetic acid to pyruvic acid.
    c. increasing the rate of fat metabolism.
    d. reducing the rate of protein metabolism.

    b

13. It is generally believed that the bulk of the oxygen debt or excess post-exercise oxygen consumption (EPOC) is due to
    a. lactic acid conversion to glycogen in the liver.
    b. gluconeogenesis.
    c. restoration of muscle CP, blood and muscle oxygen stores, and elevated tissue metabolism.
    d. None of the above are correct.

    c

14. The oxygen debt is generally higher following heavy exercise when compared to light exercise because
    a. heavy exercise produces more lactic acid.
    b. heavy exercise results in greater body heat gained, greater CP depleted, higher blood levels of epinephrine and norepinephrine, and greater depletion of blood and muscle oxygen stores.
    c. heavy exercise results in a greater level of liver glycogen depletion.
    d. heavy exercise is of shorter duration than light exercise.

    b

15. Depletion of muscle glycogen during exercise would result in
    a. an increase in fat metabolism.
    b. a decrease in fat metabolism due to a reduction in Krebs cycle intermediates.
    c. an increased rate of lactate production.
    d. None of the above are correct.

    b

16. Removal of lactic acid following a bout of intense exercise is
    a. more rapid if the subject rests compared to performing light exercise.
    b. more rapid if the subject performs heavy exercise (i.e. > 70% $\dot{V}O_2$ max) compared to rest.
    c. more rapid if the subject performs light exercise (i.e. ~ 30% $\dot{V}O_2$ max) compared to rest.
    d. None of the above are correct.

    c

17. The slow rise in oxygen uptake over time during high-intensity prolonged exercise is due to
    a. high blood levels of lactic acid.
    b. rising body temperature.
    c. rising blood levels of epinephrine and norepinephrine
    d. Both (b) and (c) are correct.

    d

Suggested Lab Experiences

Several laboratory experiences could be employed to improve students' understanding of exercise metabolism. Suggested lab experiences include:

1. *Measurement of oxygen deficit and debt.* The objective is to measure the oxygen deficit and debt during two levels of muscular exercise: (1) light exercise and (2) moderate exercise. Measurements include oxygen uptake, heart rate, and ventilation at rest, in the transition from rest-to-work, and during recovery from exercise.
2. *Determination of the lactate threshold.* The objective is to measure the change in blood lactate concentration during incremental exercise to determine the lactate threshold.

Chapter 5 Hormonal Responses to Exercise

Lecture Outline

Key Points	*Subpoints*	*Examples*
Concept of hormone-receptor interaction	Some hormones can circulate to all tissues, while affecting only a few	Thyroid-stimulating hormone
Hormone concentration determines effect on tissue	1. Rate of secretion of hormone	Control of insulin secretion
	2. Rate of inactivation of hormone	Excretion in urine
	3. Transport in plasma	Steroid hormones
	4. Plasma volume changes	Loss of plasma volume increases hormone concentration
Hormone-receptor interaction	1. Membrane transport	Insulin
	2. Stimulation of DNA	Thyroid hormones
	3. Hormone doesn't enter cell: second messenger	Cyclic AMP; calcium/calmodulin; phospholipase C
Hypothalamus and pituitary control of hormone secretion	1. Role of releasing factors on pituitary secretions	Growth hormone
	2. Effect of pituitary hormones on other glands	ACTH and cortisol release from adrenal cortex
	3. Hormones, sites of release, and principal effect	Use table of hormones and figures in text to illustrate points
Abuse of anabolic steroids and growth hormone by athletes	Normal effects vs. pathological changes	Anabolic steroids and women; growth hormone and acromegaly

Key Points	*Subpoints*	*Examples*
Hormonal control of muscle glycogen mobilization	1. Role of catecholamines 2. Calcium/calmodulin	Beta receptor and cyclic AMP Block catecholamines and effects occur; glycogen depleted only from active muscles
Control of blood glucose concentration during exercise	1. Processes involved	Glucose mobilization from liver; FFA mobilization; gluconeogenesis; blocking use of glucose
	2. Slow-acting (permissive) hormones	Summarize effects of cortisol, thyroxine, and growth hormone, but emphasize slow or permissive effect; show changes during exercise
	3. Fast-acting hormones	Summarize the effects of insulin, epinephrine, norepinephrine, and glucagon and show changes during exercise
Interaction of hormones and substrates on the mobilization of FFA during exercise	Effect of lactate on the mobilization of FFA from adipose tissue	Show figure in which lactate produced in exercise interferes with mobilization of FFA

Exam Questions

1. Place the letter of the hormone in the second column with the gland in the first column:

Name of Gland		**Hormone**
b	anterior pituitary	a. epinephrine
g	thyroid	b. growth hormone
c	adrenal cortex	c. aldosterone
h	testes	d. estrogen
d	ovaries	e. insulin
f	posterior pituitary	f. antidiuretic hormone
e	pancreas	g. T_3
a	adrenal medulla	h. testosterone

2. While hormones circulate to all tissues, some affect only a few tissues. This is due to
   a. the differences between hormones.
   b. the training state of the subject.
   c. the type of receptor at the tissue.
   d. the concentration of the hormone.

   c

3. The concentration of a hormone can be increased by
   a. decreasing the rate at which it is metabolized.
   b. increasing the number of receptors.
   c. increasing the rate at which it is excreted.
   d. All of the above are correct.

   a

4. When adenylate cyclase is activated by a hormone, the concentration of cyclic AMP increases in the cell even though the hormone does not enter the cell.
   a. true
   b. false

   a

5. Steroid hormones exert their action by
   a. activating adenyl cyclase.
   b. stimulating DNA.
   c. blocking the effect of cyclic AMP.
   d. causing an inflammation response.

   b

6. If growth hormone is secreted (or injected) in large quantities into an adult, it will result in
   a. an increase in height.
   b. diabetic-like symptoms.
   c. acromegaly.
   d. Both (b) and (c) are correct.

   d

7. If the thyroid gland does not produce a sufficient amount of T_3 or T_4, the resting metabolic rate will
   a. increase.
   b. decrease.
   c. remain the same.
   d. not change, since T_3 and T_4 do not affect the metabolic rate.

   b

8. The decrease in plasma volume and the increase in the osmolality of the plasma during exercise results in what change in antidiuretic hormone?
   a. an increase
   b. a decrease
   c. no change

   a

9. Given the importance of maintaining the plasma glucose concentration during exercise, what should happen to insulin secretion during exercise? It should
   a. increase.
   b. decrease.

   b

10. A hormone that is released from the pancreas at a higher rate during exercise to mobilize liver glucose and adipose tissue fatty acids is
    a. glucagon.
    b. somatostatin.
    c. insulin.

    a

11. The term describing the cessation of the menstrual cycle in some female athletes is
    a. dysmenorrhea.
    b. eumenorrhea.
    c. amenorrhea.

    c

12. When a drug is given to block the adrenergic receptors during exercise, muscle glycogen utilization is reduced.
    a. true
    b. false
    b

13. Given the fact that glycogen is mobilized and utilized in active muscles at a faster rate than resting muscles, what is the primary intramuscular factor driving this process?
    a. H^+
    b. Ca^{++}
    c. K^+
    d. Cl^-
    b

14. Which of the following hormones is believed to exert a "permissive" effect on the mobilization of glucose from liver and FFA from adipose tissue?
    a. epinephrine
    b. T_3 and T_4
    c. insulin
    d. glucagon
    b

15. During exercise of about 40% $\dot{V}O_2$ max, the concentration of plasma cortisol
    a. increases.
    b. decreases.
    c. remains the same.
    b

16. What happens to the concentration of plasma growth hormone during increasingly intense exercise that favors the mobilization of FFA and reduces tissue use of blood glucose?
    a. increases
    b. decreases
    c. remains the same
    a

17. What is the effect of training on the sympathetic nervous system's response to a fixed submaximal work rate?
    a. increases
    b. decreases
    c. remains the same
    b

18. Even though the concentration of insulin decreases during exercise, the muscle can still take up large quantities of plasma glucose. This is due, in part, to the recruitment of more glucose transporters.
    a. true
    b. false
    a

19. The changes in the plasma concentration of most of the hormones during maximal exercise would stimulate fatty acid mobilization from adipose tissue. However, the plasma free fatty acid concentration actually decreases. Why does this occur?
    a. fatty acid supply is depleted
    b. hormones are ineffective in maximal work
    c. lactic acid interferes with fatty acid mobilization
    d. All of the above are correct.
    c

Chapter 6 Measurement of Work, Power, and Energy Expenditure

Lecture Outline

Key Points	*Subpoints*	*Examples*
Work and power defined	1. W = F × D	5-kg weight lifted vertically 2 meters: W = 5 kp times 2m = 10 kpm
	2. P = W/T	2,000 kpm of work performed in sixty seconds: P = 2,000 kpm/60s = 33.33 kpm • s^{-1}
Measurement of work and power	1. Bench stepping	70-kg subject steps up 0.5 m bench at thirty steps/min for 10 min: W = 70 kg times 150 m = 10,500 kpm
	2. Cycle ergometer	1-min exercise @ fifty rpm (1 rev = 6m) with 1-kg resistance: W = 300 m times 1 kg = 300 kpm
	3. Treadmill	(remember that vertical displacement = % grade × D): 70-kg subject running for ten min at 200 m/min up a 7.5% grade: W = 70 kp × 150 m = 10,500 kpm
Measurement of energy expenditure	1. Direct calorimetry	Calorimeter
	2. Indirect calorimetry	Open-circuit spirometry
	3. Estimation of energy expenditure—using O_2 cost of activities	Subject runs a mile and consumes a total of 20 liter/O_2: Estimated energy expenditure = 20 1 O_2 × 5 kcal/1 O_2 = 100 kcal

Key Points	*Subpoints*	*Examples*
Calculation of exercise efficiency	1. Movement speed and efficiency—optimum speed exists for any given work rate 2. Measurement of the O_2 cost of running at various horizontal treadmill speeds offers a means of comparing running economy between individuals	efficiency = work output/energy expended × 100

Exam Questions

1. Work is defined as
   a. the ability to transform energy from one state to another.
   b. the ability to utilize oxygen.
   c. force times distance.
   d. distance times power output.
   c

2. Power is defined as
   a. the ability to perform work.
   b. work divided by time.
   c. work times force.
   d. force times distance.
   b

3. Compute the total amount of work performed in five minutes of cycle ergometer exercise in the following example.
   Given: pedalling rate = 60 rpm (6 meters per revolution)
   1.5 kg resistance against the flywheel
   The amount of work performed was
   a. 2,700 kpm.
   b. 540 kpm.
   c. 90 kpm.
   d. None of the above are correct.
   a

4. Calculate the average power output during ten minutes of cycle ergometer exercise in which a total of 7,500 kpm of work was performed.
   a. 75 kpm/min
   b. 7.5 kpm/min
   c. 750 kpm
   d. None of the above are correct.
   c

5. Calculate the amount of work performed during one minute of treadmill exercise by a 60-kg subject running at 180 meters/min up a 5% grade.
   a. 10,800 kpm
   b. 540 kpm
   c. 54 kpm
   d. 300 kpm
   b

6. Direct calorimetry is a means of determining energy expenditure and involves the measurement of
   a. metabolic oxygen consumption.
   b. metabolic heat production.
   c. ATP hydrolysis.
   d. carbon dioxide production.
   b

7. Indirect calorimetry is a technique for metabolic rate measurement and involves the measurement of
   a. metabolic heat production.
   b. total sweat rate.
   c. metabolic oxygen consumption.
   d. None of above are correct.
   c

8. The most common technique used to measure oxygen consumption in exercise physiology laboratories is
   a. closed-circuit spirometry.
   b. open-circuit spirometry.
   c. direct calorimetry.
   d. computer calorimetry.
   b

9. A MET is defined as
   a. a metabolic equivalent and is equal to resting $\dot{V}O_2$.
   b. a metabolic equivalent and is equal to 50% of resting $\dot{V}O_2$.
   c. a metabolic equivalent and is equal to 200% of resting $\dot{V}O_2$.
   d. None of the above are correct.
   a

10. Gross efficiency is defined as
   a. work output/energy expended at rest times 100%.
   b. work performed/energy expended at rest times 100%.
   c. work output/energy expended times 100%.
   d. None of above are correct.
   c

11. Calculate gross efficiency given:
   work output = 600 kpm
   energy expenditure = 7.5 kcal
   In this example, gross efficiency is equal to
   a. 1.87%.
   b. 20%.
   c. 18.7%.
   d. 15%.
   c

12. Compute oxygen consumption given:
   V_ESTPD = 50 liters/min
   $F_IO_2 = .2093$
   $F_EO_2 = .1630$
   $F_ECO_2 = .0419$
   In this example, $\dot{V}O_2$ equals
   a. 2.51 liters/min.
   b. 2.88 liters/min.
   c. 2.31 liters/min.
   d. 1.98 liters/min.
   c

13. Using the variables in question 12, compute the respiratory quotient.
   a. R = .88.
   b. R = .91.
   c. R = 1.0.
   d. R = .70.
   b

14. Recent evidence suggests that the optimum speed of movement
   a. increases as the power output increases.
   b. decreases as the power output increases.
   c. remains constant as the power output increases.
   d. None of the above are correct.
   a

15. A subject performing a 10-MET activity would have an oxygen consumption of approximately
    a. 35 ml • kg^{-1} • min^{-1}.
    b. 25 ml • kg^{-1} • min^{-1}.
    c. 45 ml • kg^{-1} • min^{-1}.
    d. 10 ml • kg^{-1} • min^{-1}.
    a

Suggested Lab Experiences

Several laboratory experiences could be employed to improve students' understanding of the measurement of work and power output during exercise. Suggested lab experiences include:

1. *Measurement of work and power output.* The objective is to measure work and power output on the cycle ergometer, during bench stepping, and during uphill treadmill exercise.
2. *Measurement of exercise efficiency.* The objective is to measure gross efficiency during submaximal cycle ergometer exercise.

Chapter 7 The Nervous System: Structure and Control of Movement

Lecture Outline

Key Points	*Subpoints*	*Examples*
General nervous system functions	1. Control of internal environment 2. Voluntary control of movement 3. Programming of spinal cord reflexes 4. Assimilation of experiences necessary for memory and learning	Temperature regulation
Organization of the nervous system	1. Central nervous system 2. Peripheral nervous system	
Structure of the neuron	1. Cell body 2. Dendrites 3. Axon	
Electrical activity in neurons	1. Resting membrane potential 2. Action potential 3. All-or-none law 4. Neurotransmitters and synaptic transmission	e.g., -70 mv EPSPs and IPSPs
Somatic receptors and reflexes	1. Kinesthetic receptors 2. Reflexes	Free nerve endings, Golgi-type receptors, and pacinian corpuscles Withdrawal reflex

Key Points	*Subpoints*	*Examples*
Vestibular apparatus and equilibrium	Organ located in inner ear—functions to maintain general equilibrium	Provides information about angular and linear acceleration
Motor functions of brain	1. Brain stem—consists of medulla, pons, and midbrain 2. Cerebrum—contains motor cortex: functions to organize complex movements, stores learned experiences, and receives sensory information 3. Cerebellum—aids in control of movement in response to feedback from proprioceptors	Controls eye movement, muscle tone; functions in equilibrium and reflexes
Motor functions of spinal cord	Spinal reflexes aid in control of movement	Spinal tuning provides the details of complex movement to assist higher brain centers in completion of a task
Control of motor functions	1. First step in motor control begins in subcortical and cortical areas, which signal association areas of the cortex to form a "rough draft" of the planned movement 2. The cerebellum and basal ganglia then convert the rough draft into a precise temporal and spatial excitation program	

Key Points	*Subpoints*	*Examples*
Autonomic nervous system	1. Important role in maintaining the constancy of internal environment	
	2. Autonomic nervous system is divided into two divisions:	
	(a) Sympathetic nervous system	Epinephrine and norepinephrine are released at the effector organ
	(b) Parasympathetic nervous system	Acetylcholine is released at the effector organ

Exam Questions

1. Anatomically, the nervous system can be divided into two main parts:
   a. afferent and efferent.
   b. central nervous system and peripheral nervous system.
   c. neurons and synapses.
   d. None of the above are correct.
   b

2. Nerve fibers that conduct impulses away from the central nervous system are called
   a. efferent.
   b. afferent.
   c. dendrites.
   d. None of the above are correct.
   a

3. Neurons can be divided into three basic parts:
   a. cell body, soma, and axon.
   b. soma, dendrites, and Schwann cells.
   c. cell body, dendrites, and axon.
   d. afferent, efferent, and dendrites.
   c

4. Neurons are negatively charged on the inside of the cell with respect to the charge on the exterior of the cell. This electrical charge difference is called
   a. irritability.
   b. conductivity.
   c. action potential.
   d. resting membrane potential.
   d

5. The action potential or nerve impulse is achieved by
   a. sodium gates opening and allowing a rapid entry of sodium ions.
   b. the exit of chloride from the neuron.
   c. the entry of potassium into the cell.
   d. None of the above are correct.
   a

6. Nerve fibers that carry impulses toward the central nervous system are called
   a. efferent fibers.
   b. dendrites.
   c. afferent fibers.
   d. None of the above are correct.
   c

7. Receptors that are responsible for position "sense" are termed
   a. efferent fibers.
   b. proprioceptors.
   c. free nerve endings.
   d. None of the above are correct.

   b

8. The _____ is an organ located in the inner ear and is responsible for maintaining general equilibrium.
   a. pacinian corpuscle
   b. Golgi tendon organ
   c. vestibular apparatus
   d. None of the above are correct.

   c

9. The brain stem is located just above the spinal cord and contains
   a. the medulla, pons, and midbrain.
   b. cerebellum, pons, and medulla.
   c. basal ganglia and medulla.
   d. None of the above are correct.

   a

10. The motor cortex is concerned with voluntary movement and is located within
    a. the cerebellum.
    b. the cerebrum.
    c. the brain stem.
    d. the hypothalamus.

    b

11. The area of the brain that aids in control of movement and may initiate fast ballistic movements is the
    a. cerebrum.
    b. motor cortex.
    c. brain stem.
    d. cerebellum.

    d

12. Voluntary movements are planned and executed by the motor cortex without outside influence from other areas of the nervous system.
    a. true
    b. false

    b

13. The autonomic nervous system can be divided into two functional and anatomical divisions called
    a. sympathetic and unsympathetic.
    b. sympathetic and parasympathetic.
    c. afferent and efferent.
    d. CNA and peripheral.

    b

14. The principal role of the autonomic nervous system is to maintain the constancy of the body's internal environment.
    a. true
    b. false

    a

15. An excitatory neurotransmitter results in
    a. increased neuronal permeability to sodium and results in IPSPs.
    b. increased neuronal permeability to sodium and results in EPSPs.
    c. increased neuronal permeability to potassium and results in IPSPs.
    d. increased neuronal permeability to potassium and results in IPSPs.

    b

16. Parkinson's disease is a disorder of the basal ganglia resulting in
    a. an impairment in maximal speed of movement.
    b. increased involuntary movement of tremors.
    c. an impairment in hearing.
    d. impaired reaction times.

    b

17. The term *kinesthesia* refers to
    a. the study of movement.
    b. the study of exercise.
    c. conscious recognition of the position of body parts with respect to each other.
    d. none of the above.
    c

Suggested Lab Experiences

Several laboratory experiences could be employed to improve students' understanding of the nervous system. Most laboratory experiments in neurophysiology require sophisticated and expensive equipment that often does not exist in exercise physiology laboratories. However, a simple suggested lab experience in neurophysiology is:

1. *Demonstration of the stretch reflex.* The objective is to demonstrate the stretch reflex by tapping on the patellar tendon with a rubber mallet.

Chapter 8 Skeletal Muscle: Structure and Function

Lecture Outline

Key Points	*Subpoints*	*Examples*
Structure of skeletal muscle	1. Skeletal muscle is composed of several types of tissue: (a) muscle cells, (b) connective tissue, (c) blood, and (d) nerve tissue 2. Three layers of connective tissue surround muscle: (a) epimysium (b) perimysium (c) endomysium 3. Myofibrils contain two principal types of protein: (a) actin, (b) myosin 4. Troponin and tropomyosin act as regulatory proteins in the control of contraction	Thin-twisted filament Heavy-large filament Ca^{++} binds to troponin to initiate the contractile process
Neuromuscular junction	1. Release of acetylcholine at neuromuscular junction results in an end-plate potential and the eventual release of Ca^{++} from the SR 2. A motor neuron and all muscle cells that it innervates are called a motor unit	

Key Points	*Subpoints*	*Examples*
Muscular contraction	Overview of sliding filament theory: shortening of myofibrils occurs due to myosin cross-bridges extending to actin and pulling the actin molecule over the myosin	
Energy for contraction	ATP provides the needed energy for contraction	
Regulation of contraction	Troponin and tropomyosin act as regulatory proteins	
Isometric and isotonic contractions	1. Isometric contractions result in muscle tension increasing, but joint angle does not change	
	2. Isotonic contractions result in an increase in muscle tension and a change in joint angle	
Fiber types	1. Fast-twitch fibers—contain relatively few mitochondria, high ATPase activity, and fatigue rapidly	"white muscle"
	2. Slow-twitch fibers—contain high numbers of mitochondria, low ATPase activity, and are fatigue-resistant	"red muscle"
	3. Intermediate fibers—contain biochemical and mechanical characteristics that are somewhere between fast-twitch and slow-twitch fibers	

Key Points	*Subpoints*	*Examples*
Muscle as a plastic tissue	Muscle composition is moldable in response to changes in physical activity Strength training results in an increase in muscle size and strength Endurance training results in no increase in muscle size or strength but results in increases in muscle oxidative capacity	
Fiber types and performance	The percentage of fast- and slow-twitch fibers found in an athlete may play an important role in determining success in certain sports	Successful sprinters generally possess a large percentage of fast-twitch fibers Successful distance runners generally possess a high percentage of slow-twitch fibers
Force regulation in muscle	Amount of force exerted during muscular contraction is dependent on the types and numbers of motor units recruited, the initial length of the muscle, and the nature of the neural stimulation of the motor units	The effect of the number of motor units recruited on force production can be demonstrated by increasing the amount of stimulation applied to an isolated muscle preparation The influence of muscle length on force production is linked to the overlap between actin and myosin A tetanic contraction results in greater force production than a simple twitch

Key Points	*Subpoints*	*Examples*
Force-velocity relationship	1. Peak force generated by a muscle decreases as the speed of movement increases 2. At any given speed of movement, the peak force exerted by muscle is greater in a muscle that has a high percentage of fast-twitch fibers when compared to a muscle that contains a high percentage of slow-twitch fibers	Greatest amount of force is generated at slow speeds
Power-velocity relationships	1. The peak power generated by any muscle increases up to a movement speed of 200–400 degrees/s; at speeds above 400 degrees/s there is a plateau in power output due to the decrease in muscular force 2. At any given velocity of movement, peak power generated is greater in muscle that contains a high percentage of fast-twitch fibers when compared to a muscle that contains a high percentage of slow-twitch fibers	

Key Points	*Subpoints*	*Examples*
Receptors in muscle	1. Muscle spindle functions as a length detector (intrafusal fibers are innervated by gamma motor neurons)—muscle spindles contain two types of nerve endings: (a) primary (respond to dynamic changes in length) and (b) secondary (provides continuous information concerning static length of muscle)	Responsible for the stretch reflex
	2. Golgi tendon organs monitor muscular tension	Act as a safety device to prevent injury
	3. Muscle chemoreceptors respond to changes in local pH and metabolite concentrations	Free nerve endings

Exam Questions

1. The layer of connective tissue that surrounds the outside of skeletal muscle (i.e., just below the fascia) is called the
   a. epimysium.
   b. perimysium.
   c. endomysium.
   d. None of the above are correct.
   a

2. The cell membrane around muscle is called the
   a. soma.
   b. plasma membrane.
   c. mucous membrane.
   d. sarcolemma.
   d

3. The two principal contractile proteins found in skeletal muscle are
   a. actin and troponin.
   b. actin and myosin.
   c. troponin and tropomyosin.
   d. myosin and tropomyosin.
   b

4. Calcium is stored in muscle within the
   a. Golgi organs.
   b. H zone.
   c. sarcoplasmic reticulum.
   d. None of the above are correct.
   c

5. The trigger to initiate the contractile process in skeletal muscle is
   a. potassium binding to myosin.
   b. calcium binding to tropomyosin.
   c. calcium binding to troponin.
   d. ATP binding to the myosin cross-bridges.

   c

6. A muscular contraction that results in a movement of body parts is called a
   a. isometric contraction.
   b. static contraction.
   c. isotonic or dynamic contraction.
   d. muscle twitch.

   c

7. Fast-twitch fibers contain
   a. relatively large number of mitochondria and low ATPase activity.
   b. a relatively small number of mitochondria and low ATPase activity.
   c. a relatively small number of mitochondria and high ATPase activity.
   d. None of the above are correct.

   c

8. The motor neuron and all the muscle fibers it innervates is called a
   a. motor junction.
   b. motor unit.
   c. motor end plate.
   d. None of the above are correct.

   b

9. The site where the motor neuron and muscle cell meet is called the
   a. end-plate potential.
   b. motor unit.
   c. sarcolemma.
   d. None of the above are correct.

   d

10. The breakdown of ATP in muscle is accomplished via the enzyme
    a. lactate dehydrogenase.
    b. succinate dehydrogenase.
    c. ATPase.
    d. phosphofructokinase.

    c

11. Skeletal muscle fibers that contain large numbers of mitochondria and myoglobin would likely be classified as slow-twitch (i.e., oxidative) or type I fibers.
    a. true
    b. false

    a

12. High activities of the enzyme ATPase are found in both slow-twitch and fast-twitch fibers.
    a. true
    b. false

    b

13. Successful endurance athletes generally possess
    a. a high percentage of slow-twitch fibers.
    b. a high percentage of intermediate fibers.
    c. a high percentage of fast-twitch fibers.
    d. an equal percentage of slow-twitch and fast-twitch fiber.

    a

14. The amount of force exerted during muscular contraction is dependent upon
    a. the type of motor units recruited and nothing else.
    b. the type of motor units recruited, the initial length of the muscle, and the nature of the neural stimulation.
    c. the length of the muscle fibers only.
    d. None of the above are correct.

    b

15. At any given velocity of movement, the peak force is greater in muscles that contain a high percentage of fast-twitch fibers when compared to muscles that possess predominantly slow-twitch fibers.
    a. true
    b. false
    a

16. Muscle spindles provide sensory information relative to
    a. the amount of force generated by muscle during a contraction.
    b. the length of muscle.
    c. the amount of energy expended during a contraction.
    d. None of the above are correct.
    b

17. The thin muscle cells located within the muscle spindle are called
    a. extrafusal fibers.
    b. gamma fibers.
    c. intrafusal fibers.
    d. None of the above are correct.
    c

18. The "knee jerk" or stretch reflex is due to rapid stretch of the Golgi tendon organ, which results in a reflex contraction of the extensor muscles.
    a. true
    b. false
    b

19. The Golgi tendon organs monitor
    a. tension produced by muscular contraction.
    b. the length of muscle.
    c. the concentration of sodium ions in the sarcoplasm.
    d. the position of joints during movement.
    a

20. Recent evidence suggests that rigorous exercise training can result in a conversion of muscle fiber type.
    a. true
    b. false
    a

Suggested Lab Experiences

Several laboratory experiences could be employed to improve students' understanding of muscular function during exercise. Suggested lab experiences include:

1. *Demonstration of force-velocity and power-velocity relationships.* The objective of this laboratory experience is to demonstrate the influence of movement speed on force and power production. Measurement of force and power output (i.e., requires an isokinetic device) using the leg extensors at various speeds can be used to demonstrate the graphic relationship between movement speed and the generation of force/power output.
2. *Demonstration of stretch reflex.* The objective is to demonstrate the response of the muscle spindle to a rapid change in muscle length. The "knee jerk" response can be demonstrated by tapping the patellar tendon with a rubber mallet.

3. *Demonstration of the impact of muscle length on tension development.* The objective is to demonstrate the influence of muscle length on the development of tension. This laboratory requires the use of an in vitro isolated muscle preparation (e.g., frog or rat muscle). A micrometer can be used to alter muscle length while tension development (at a voltage that will elicit a maximal twitch) is monitored with a pressure transducer.

Chapter 9 Circulatory Adaptations to Exercise

Lecture Outline

Key Points	*Subpoints*	*Examples*
Organization of the circulatory system	1. Closed loop—circulates blood to all tissues 2. Two circuits—systemic and pulmonary 3. Systemic blood flows away from the heart and begins in the aorta with the flow sequence being from arteries to arterioles to capillaries to venules to veins then back to right side of heart 4. All exchange of gases and nutrients occurs within capillaries	
Structure of the heart	1. Four chambers—two pumps-in-on	Systemic and pulmonary circuits
	2. Right and left AV valves prevent backflow into the atria	Right AV valve is called the tricuspid Left AV valve is called the bicuspid or mitral valve
	3. Right and left semilunar valves prevent backflow into the ventricles	Right semilunar valve is called the pulmonary semilunar valve Left semilunar valve is called the aortic semilunar valve

Key Points	*Subpoints*	*Examples*
Heart: myocardium and cardiac cycle	1. The heart wall is composed of three layers: (a) epicardium, (b) myocardium, and the (c) endocardium	
	2. Cardiac cycle consists of two phases: (a) systole and (b) diastole	At rest: systole = 0.3 s; diastole = 0.5 s; Total time = 0.8 s
	3. Arterial blood pressure can be estimated via a sphygmomanometer	e.g., male resting BP = 120/80 female resting BP = 110/70
	4. Hypertension is classified into two categories: (a) primary or (b) secondary	Resting BP > 140/90 is considered to be indicative of hypertension
Electrical activity of the heart	1. Electrical activity of the heart can be monitored using an electrocardiogram (ECG)	ECG pattern is represented by the P, QRS, and T waves
	2. Sinoatrial (SA) node is the normal cardiac pacemaker	
	3. The atrioventricular (AV) node conducts the electrical impulse from the atria to the ventricles	
Cardiac output	1. $\dot{Q}$ = HR times SV	21-year-old male: Rest $\dot{Q}$ ~5 l/min HR = ~ 72 BPM SV = ~ 70 ml/beat
	2. Venous return during exercise ultimately determines $\dot{Q}$. Venous return during exercise is increased by: (a) venoconstriction, (b) mechanical pumping action of muscles, and the (c) respiratory pump	21-year-old female: Rest $\dot{Q}$ = ~ 4.5 l/min HR = ~ 75 BPM SV = ~ 60 ml/beat

Key Points	*Subpoints*	*Examples*
Regulation of heart rate	1. Cardiovascular control center is located in the medulla oblongata 2. HR is increased by sympathetic outflow to the heart 3. HR is decreased by parasympathetic outflow to the heart	Cardiac accelerator nerves Vagus nerve
Regulation of stroke volume	SV is regulated by three variables: (a) end-diastolic volume; (b) aortic pressure; and (c) strength of ventricular contraction	Frank-Starling law—Increase in EDV results in increased SV
Blood composition	1. Blood composed of: (a) plasma and (b) cells 2. Hematocrit is defined as the ratio of RBC volume to total blood volume	RBCs are the most numerous cells in blood Typical male Hct = 42% Female Hct = 38%
Relationships between pressure, resistance, and flow	1. Blood flow is proportional to D P/R R = length times viscosity/radius^4 2. Arterioles offer the greatest source of vascular resistance	
Changes in oxygen delivery to muscle during exercise	1. Increased O_2 delivery to muscle during exercise is accomplished by increasing $\dot{Q}$ and causing a redistribution of blood flow to the contracting skeletal muscle 2. Blood flow to the gut decreases as a linear function of work rate above 50% $\dot{V}O_2$ max	During max exercise up to 80% of total $\dot{Q}$ is directed toward the working muscles

Key Points	*Subpoints*	*Examples*
Changes in cardiac output during exercise	1. $\dot{Q}$ increases as a linear function of the metabolic rate during exercise 2. SV increases up to ~ 40% $\dot{V}O_2$ max during exercise, with any additional increases in Q being due to increases in HR 3. Max HR declines with age	Max HR = 220 - age
Changes in arterial-mixed venous O_2 content during exercise	1. a-$\bar{v}O_2$ difference represents the amount of O_2 that is taken up and used by the tissues 2. The a-$\bar{v}O_2$ difference increases as a function of the metabolic rate during exercise	
Regulation of local blood flow during exercise	1. Muscle as well as other body tissues have the ability to regulate blood flow in direct proportion to their metabolic need 2. At the beginning of exercise, withdrawal of sympathetic stimulation of arterioles results in an increase in muscle blood flow 3. After this initial sympathetic withdrawal, local factors (K^+, ADP, H^+ etc.) work together to maintain muscle blood in proportion to the metabolic need	Occurs rapidly after exercise begins

Key Points	*Subpoints*	*Examples*
Circulatory responses to exercise	1. Emotional influence—apprehension and/or fear can influence the HR/BP response to submaximal exercise	
	2. HR increases rapidly in the transition from rest to work reaching a steady-state within two to three minutes	
	3. HR and BP decline rapidly during recovery from exercise—speed of recovery is dependent on the intensity and duration of exercise and fitness level of subject	
	4. HR and MAP increase as a linear function of the metabolic rate during incremental exercise	Graded stress test
	5. At any given metabolic rate, both HR and BP are higher during arm work when compared to leg work	Arm ergometry vs. leg ergometry
	6. The extent of HR recovery during intermittent exercise depends on the exercising environment, subject fitness, and the intensity/duration of the exercise	Interval training
	7. HR may drift upward (CV drift) during prolonged exercise in a hot/humid environment	Marathons run in hot weather may result in competitors running at maximal HRs for most of the event

Key Points	*Subpoints*	*Examples*
Regulation of cardiovascular adjustments to exercise	1. Central command theory probably explains much of the CV changes at the onset of exercise 2. Muscle chemoreceptors, mechanoreceptors, and baroreceptors may also contribute to the "total" CV adjustment to exercise	

Exam Questions

1. The primary role of the cardiovascular system is to
   a. convey heat away from deep body tissues.
   b. deliver adequate amounts of oxygen and remove wastes from body tissues.
   c. serve as a buffer fluid for metabolic wastes during exercise.
   d. None of the above are correct.
   b

2. In order to meet the increased oxygen demands of muscle during exercise, two major adjustments in blood flow must be made:
   a. an increase in HR and blood pressure.
   b. an increase in brain blood flow and blood flow to the skin.
   c. an increase in cardiac output and a redistribution of blood flow from inactive tissues to skeletal muscles.
   d. an increase in muscle blood flow and an increase in blood flow to the liver.
   c

3. All gas exchange between the vascular system and tissues occurs in
   a. venules.
   b. capillaries.
   c. arterioles.
   d. veins.
   b

4. Backflow of blood from the arteries into the ventricles is prevented by the
   a. semilunar valves.
   b. bicuspid valve.
   c. atrioventricular valves.
   d. None of the above are correct.
   a

5. The muscle of the heart is referred to as the
   a. pericardium.
   b. myocardium.
   c. epicardium.
   d. endocardium.
   b

6. Electrical impulses are conducted between heart muscle cells by
   a. intercalated discs.
   b. intermediate junctions.
   c. minute synapses of the sympathetic nervous system.
   d. None of the above are correct.

   a

7. The contraction phase of the heart is called
   a. diastole.
   b. atrial contraction.
   c. systole.
   d. None of the above are correct.

   c

8. In a healthy heart the time spent in systole is generally
   a. longer than diastole.
   b. equal to diastole.
   c. shorter than diastole.
   d. three times longer than diastole.

   c

9. During exercise, the time spent in diastole and systole
   a. remains unchanged.
   b. is decreased equally.
   c. is decreased with the greatest decrease occurring in diastole.
   d. is increased.

   c

10. The difference between systolic and diastolic blood pressure is called
    a. the pulse pressure.
    b. mean arterial blood pressure.
    c. the brachial pressure.
    d. None of the above are correct.

    a

11. The normal pacemaker of the heart is the
    a. atrioventricular node.
    b. sinoatrial node.
    c. AV node.
    d. SV node.

    b

12. The _____ represents ventricular repolarization during a recording of the electrical activity (i.e., ECG) of the heart.
    a. P wave
    b. QRS complex
    c. T wave
    d. R wave

    c

13. The three principal mechanisms for increasing venous return during exercise are
    a. an increase in stroke volume, HR, and compliance of the vascular system.
    b. venoconstriction, pumping action of muscle, and the pumping action of the respiratory system.
    c. an increase in vascular resistance, an increase in HR, and a decrease in blood pressure.
    d. None of the above are correct.

    b

14. An increase in parasympathetic outflow to the heart results in
    a. an increase in HR.
    b. a decrease in HR.
    c. a slight increase in arterial blood pressure.
    d. a slight decrease in arterial blood pressure followed by an increase in HR.

    b

15. The cardiovascular control center is located in
    a. the medulla oblongata.
    b. carotid sinus.
    c. cerebrum.
    d. atria of the heart.

    a

16. The fact that an increase in end-diastolic ventricular volume increases the stroke volume of the heart is an illustration of
    a. the influence of the parasympathetic nervous system on cardiac output.
    b. the Frank-Starling law of the heart.
    c. the influence of atrioventricular node on cardiac output.
    d. None of the above are correct.
    b

17. The increase in cardiac output that occurs during exercise is due to
    a. both an increase in mean arterial pressure and a decrease in vascular resistance.
    b. a decrease in vascular resistance only.
    c. an increase in mean arterial blood pressure only.
    d. an increase in heart rate and a decrease in mean arterial blood pressure.
    a

18. The most important variable that determines resistance to blood flow is
    a. the viscosity of blood.
    b. the length of the blood vessel.
    c. the diameter of the vessel.
    d. None of the above are correct.
    c

19. The relationship between cardiac output and metabolic rate is
    a. linear.
    b. curvilinear.
    c. exponential.
    d. None of the above are correct.
    a

20. Stroke volume continues to increase during exercise up to approximately
    a. 20% of $\dot{V}O_2$ max.
    b. 30% of $\dot{V}O_2$ max.
    c. 40% of $\dot{V}O_2$ max.
    d. 60% of $\dot{V}O_2$ max.
    c

21. The decrease in maximal heart rate with age can be estimated via
    a. HR max = 220 - age.
    b. HR max = 200 - age.
    c. HR max = 210 - age.
    d. HR max = 205 - age.
    a

22. Autoregulation of local blood flow is due to
    a. the withdrawal of sympathetic impulses to arterioles.
    b. an increase in parasympathetic outflow to arterioles.
    c. local factors such as a decrease in PO_2, an increase in PCO_2, and potassium concentrations.
    d. None of the above are correct.
    c

23. In general, heart rate increases in direct proportion to the metabolic rate during exercise.
    a. true
    b. false
    a

24. Most of the increase in mean arterial blood pressure that occurs during dynamic (isotonic) incremental exercise is due to
    a. an increase in diastolic blood pressure.
    b. the increase in systolic blood pressure alone.
    c. both an increase in diastolic and systolic blood pressure.
    d. None of the above are correct.
    b

25. At any level of oxygen consumption, heart rate and blood pressure are lower during leg work when compared to arm work.
    a. true
    b. false
    a

26. The central command theory of cardiovascular control argues that the initial signal to the cardiovascular system at the beginning of exercise comes from higher brain centers.
    a. true
    b. false
    a

27. A local increase in the adenosine concentration around arterioles would result in
    a. vasoconstriction
    b. no change in vessel diameter
    c. vasodilation
    d. None of the above are correct.
    c

28. The arterial-venous oxygen difference
    a. increases as a function of exercise intensity.
    b. does not change during exercise.
    c. decreases as the exercise intensity increases.
    d. None of the above are correct.
    a

29. The relationship between oxygen uptake, cardiac output, and the arterial-venous oxygen difference is described mathematically by the
    a. Hill equation.
    b. Fenn equation.
    c. Fick equation.
    d. Frank-Starling law.
    c

30. Resistance to blood flow is
    a. directly proportional to the length of the vessel.
    b. inversely proportional to the viscosity of the blood.
    c. directly related to the diameter of the vessel.
    d. All of the above are correct.
    a

Suggested Lab Experiences

Several laboratory experiences could be employed to improve students' understanding of the cardiovascular adaptations to exercise. Suggested lab experiences include:

1. *HR and BP responses to submaximal exercise.* The objective is to measure the change in HR and BP during the transition from rest to steady-state exercise. Measurements could include HR and BP at rest and then every thirty seconds during the transition from rest to steady-state (i.e., submaximal-constant load) exercise on the cycle ergometer.
2. *HR and BP responses to incremental exercise.* The objective is to measure changes in HR and BP during incremental exercise. Estimations of $\dot{Q}$ and SV could be made following the experiment using published values for changes in the a-$\overline{v}O_2$ difference during exercise.
3. *Cardiovascular responses to arm and leg exercise.* The objective is to compare the HR and BP responses to arm and leg exercise at the same metabolic rate (i.e., arm ergometry vs. cycle ergometry).

Chapter 10 Respiration during Exercise

Lecture Outline

Key Points	*Subpoints*	*Examples*
Function of the lung	1. Primary function is to provide a means of gas exchange between environment and body 2. Secondary functions include a role in the maintenance of acid-base balance and as a reservoir for blood	Maintenance of a constant arterial PO_2 and PCO_2
Structure of the respiratory system	1. Conductive zone 2. Respiratory zone	Trachea, bronchi Alveoli
Mechanics of breathing	1. Inspiration 2. Expiration 3. Airway resistance	Major muscle: diaphragm Passive at rest Airflow = D P/R
Pulmonary ventilation	1. Anatomical dead space 2. Alveolar ventilation 3. Total minute ventilation	$\dot{V} = \dot{V}_A + \dot{V}_D$
Pulmonary volumes and capacities	1. Vital capacity 2. Residual volume 3. Total lung capacity	
Diffusion of gases	1. Dalton's law of partial pressures 2. Fick's law of diffusion	P_IO_2 = .2093 times 760 mmHg = 159 mmHg $\dot{V}$ = A/T times D times DP

Key Points	*Subpoints*	*Examples*
Ventilation-perfusion relationships	1. Blood flow to the lung is greatest in the basal regions and lowest in the apex in the upright position	Linear decrease in blood flow from the bottom to the top of the lung
	2. Regional ventilation in the lung increases from the top to the bottom of the lung	
	3. Normal gas exchange requires a matching of ventilation to perfusion	Ideal $\dot{V}/Q$ relationship = 1
	4. While light exercise may improve $\dot{V}/Q$ relationships, heavy exercise results in $\dot{V}/Q$ inequalities and may impair gas exchange.	Widening of A-a gradient during heavy exercise
O_2 and CO_2 transport in blood	1. 99% of O_2 transported via Hb	1.34 ml O_2 per gm Hb
	2. O_2-Hb dissociation curve is sigmoidal and increases sharply up to a PO_2 of 40 Torr. Above PO_2 of 40 Torr the curve rises slowly to a plateau around 90–100 Torr	
	3. O_2-Hb curve is shifted to the right by an increase in $[H^+]$, temperature and 2–3 DPG levels	Bohr effect
	4. CO_2 is transported in three forms: (a) dissolved CO_2 (10%); (b) carbamino-hemoglobin (20%); and (c) HCO_3^- (70%)	

Key Points	*Subpoints*	*Examples*
Ventilation and acid-base	Pulmonary ventilation can remove H^+ via the following reaction: $CO_2 + H_2O \rightleftharpoons H_2CO_3 \rightleftharpoons H^+ + HCO_3^-$	Hyperventilation at work rates above the lactate threshold
Ventilatory and blood gas responses to exercise	1. Ventilation increases rapidly at the onset of exercise—followed by a slower rise toward steady state	Rest-to-work transition
	2. Arterial PO_2 decreases slightly in the transition from rest-to-steady-state exercise suggesting that alveolar ventilation does not increase as rapidly as metabolism	
	3. Ventilation drifts upward during prolonged constant-load exercise	Exercise in a hot and humid environment
	4. Ventilation increases in a linear fashion during incremental exercise until the lactate threshold is reached—above which the increase is alinear with respect to $\dot{V}O_2$	Ventilatory threshold

Key Points	*Subpoints*	*Examples*
Control of ventilation	1. The respiratory control center is located in the medulla oblongata and receives input from peripheral chemoreceptors	
	2. An increase in arterial PCO_2 or a decrease in arterial PO_2 results in an increased alveolar ventilation due to peripheral chemoreceptor feedback to the respiratory control center	Acute exposure to altitude increases alveolar ventilation
	3. Three schools of thought exist concerning the control of breathing during exercise: (a) neural hypothesis; (b) humoral (CO_2 flow) hypothesis; and (c) neural-humoral hypothesis. It is commonly believed that ventilatory control occurs due to interaction of both neural and humoral input	

Exam Questions

1. The primary purpose of the pulmonary system is to
   a. regulate acid-base balance.
   b. provide an interface for gas exchange between the environment and the body.
   c. regulate cardiac output.
   d. control the bicarbonate level in the blood.
   b

2. The term *ventilation* refers to
   a. the cooling of the airways by respiration.
   b. the random movement of molecules from an area of high concentration to an area of lower concentration.
   c. the mechanical process of moving air in and out of the lungs.
   d. None of the above are correct.
   c

3. The most important muscle of inspiration is the
   a. diaphragm.
   b. rectus abdominous.
   c. internal oblique.
   d. external intercostals.
   a

4. The volume of gas that reaches the respiratory zone (gas-exchange zone) of the lung is termed
   a. anatomical dead space.
   b. minute ventilation.
   c. alveolar ventilation.
   d. None of the above are correct.
   c

5. According to Fick's law of diffusion, the rate of diffusion for a gas is greater when the surface area for diffusion is large and the "driving pressure" (i.e., partial pressure) between the two sides of tissue is high.
   a. true
   b. false
   a

6. In the standing position, considerable inequality of blood flow exists within the human lung due to
   a. partial pressure differences across the lung.
   b. differences in vascular resistance in the lateral areas of the lung.
   c. gravity.
   d. None of the above are correct.
   c

7. A ventilation-perfusion relationship in the lung of less than 0.50 would be indicative of perfect conditions for gas exchange.
   a. true
   b. false
   b

8. The major portion of O_2 that is transported in the blood is in
   a. solution as a dissolved gas.
   b. the form of oxyhemoglobin.
   c. the form of carboxyhemoglobin.
   d. the form of deoxyhemoglobin.
   b

9. In general, because of blood hemoglobin concentration differences, males transport less oxygen per unit of blood volume than females.
   a. true
   b. false
   b

10. A decrease in blood pH results in a left shift of the O_2-Hb dissociation curve and a reduced affinity for oxygen by hemoglobin.
   a. true
   b. false
   b

11. Myoglobin is a red pigment found in skeletal muscle that serves to
   a. transport CO_2 from the cell membrane to the mitochondria.
   b. transport O_2 from the cell membrane to the mitochondria.
   c. buffer changes in hydrogen ion concentration in the cell.
   d. None of the above are correct.
   b

12. Carbon dioxide is transported in the blood principally as
   a. carbamino-hemoglobin.
   b. dissolved CO_2 in solution in the blood.
   c. bicarbonate.
   d. None of the above are correct.
   c

13. An increase in alveolar ventilation serves to lower arterial PCO_2 and increase blood pH.
    a. true
    b. false
    a

14. Minute ventilation tends to "drift" upward during constant load submaximal exercise performed in a hot and humid environment due to an increase in blood temperature.
    a. true
    b. false
    a

15. Exercise-induced hypoxemia that may occur in elite endurance athletes during heavy exercise is likely due to
    a. overt lung disease.
    b. a reduced alveolar ventilation due to exercise-induced asthma.
    c. a right-to-left shunt.
    d. a diffusion limitation secondary to a rapid red blood cell transit time.
    d

16. The respiratory control center is located within
    a. the medulla oblongata.
    b. the cerebrum.
    c. carotid bodies.
    d. cerebellum.
    a

17. The carotid bodies are chemoreceptors that are sensitive to changes in arterial
    a. H^+ and K^+ concentrations.
    b. pH, PCO_2, and PO_2.
    c. pH and K^+ concentrations.
    d. PCO_2 and pH only.
    b

18. The ventilatory central chemoreceptors respond to changes in
    a. the pH of mixed venous blood.
    b. the pH of cerebral spinal fluid.
    c. the PO_2, pH, and PCO_2 of cerebral spinal fluid.
    d. None of the above are correct.
    b

19. A decrease in arterial PO_2 below 70 mm Hg would likely result in
    a. a decrease in alveolar ventilation.
    b. an increase in alveolar ventilation.
    c. a short breath hold followed by irregular breathing patterns.
    d. None of the above are correct.
    b

20. An increase in arterial hydrogen ion concentration (i.e., a decrease in pH) would result in a decrease in alveolar ventilation.
    a. true
    b. false
    b

21. Ventilatory control during submaximal exercise is likely due to
    a. afferent feedback to the respiratory control center.
    b. efferent neural activity from higher brain centers.
    c. humoral (blood borne) stimuli.
    d. Some combination of (a), (b), and (c) is correct.
    d

22. The alinear rise in ventilation observed during incremental exercise (i.e., ventilatory threshold) is thought to be principally due to
    a. a decrease in arterial PO_2.
    b. an increase in arterial PCO_2.
    c. an increase in arterial pH.
    d. a decrease in arterial pH.
    d

23. Activation of rectus abdominus muscles would result in
    a. active inspiration.
    b. passive inspiration.
    c. active expiration.
    d. Both (a) and (b) are correct.
    c

24. The ideal ventilation-perfusion ratio in the lung is 1.
    a. true
    b. false
    a

25. A decrease in arterial PO_2 below 70 mm Hg would increase pulmonary ventilation by stimulation of the
    a. arterial bodies.
    b. carotid bodies.
    c. central chemoreceptors.
    d. Both (a) and (c) are correct.
    b

26. In some species lung PCO_2 receptors may exist that serve to match CO_2 return to the lung with ventilation.
    a. true
    b. false
    a

27. During exercise at sea level, young healthy untrained subjects generally maintain exercise arterial PO_2 within
    a. 1 mm Hg of resting values.
    b. 10–12 mm Hg of resting values.
    c. 30–40 mm Hg of resting values.
    d. None of the above are correct.
    b

28. An increase in blood temperature would result in a left shift in the oxyhemoglobin dissociation curve.
    a. true
    b. false
    b

Suggested Lab Experiences

Several laboratory exercises could be employed to improve students' understanding of the pulmonary system during exercise. Suggested lab experiences include:

1. *Pulmonary function lab.* The objective is to demonstrate pulmonary function testing using simple spirometry or other more sophisticated pulmonary testing equipment. Measurements could include lung volumes, vital capacity, FEV_1, and diffusion.
2. *Ventilatory response to exercise.* The objective is to demonstrate the ventilatory response in the transition from rest to constant load submaximal exercise and during incremental exercise. Tests can be performed on either treadmill or cycle ergometer. Measurements could include changes in minute ventilation, tidal volume, frequency of breathing, and end tidal gas tensions.
3. *Ventilatory response to hypoxic gases and carbon dioxide.* The objective is to demonstrate the ventilatory response to hypoxia and/or hypercapnia. Measurements include changes in end tidal gas tensions and minute ventilation in response to hypoxic and hypercapnic challenges.

Chapter 11 Acid-Base Balance during Exercise

Lecture Outline

Key Points	*Subpoints*	*Examples*
Acids, bases, and pH	1. Acids are molecules that can liberate hydrogen ions	Lactic acid
	2. Bases are molecules capable of binding to hydrogen ions	Bicarbonate
	3. $pH = \log_{10}[H^+]$	Normal arterial blood $pH = 7.4$
Hydrogen ion production during exercise	1. Volatile acids	Carbon dioxide
	2. Fixed acids	Sulfuric acid
	3. Organic acids	Lactic acid produced at high work rates
Acid-base balance and the kidney	1. The kidneys do not play an important role in acid-base balance during exercise due to the time course of the renal response	
	2. Renal regulation of acid-base balance occurs via elimination or retention of hydrogen ions or bicarbonate ions	

Key Points	*Subpoints*	*Examples*
Acid-base regulation during exercise	1. Regulation of cellular pH is critical due to the influence of hydrogen ions on metabolism and muscular contraction	
	2. Buffer systems consist of a weak acid and a weak base	
	3. First line of defense in protecting against pH change during exercise is intracellular buffers	Cellular proteins and phosphate groups
	4. Blood contains three principal buffer systems: (a) proteins; (b) hemoglobin; and (c) bicarbonate	Bicarbonate is most important buffer system in body
	5. Respiratory compensation aids in elimination of $[H^+]$ during exercise	$CO_2 + H_2O \leftrightarrow H_2CO_3 \leftrightarrow H^+ + HCO_3^-$

Exam Questions

1. Acids are defined as
   a. electrolytes that release hydroxyl ions (OH^-).
   b. electrolytes that release hydrogen ions (H^+).
   c. substances that combine with electrolytes to form anions.
   d. None of the above are correct.

   b

2. A base is a molecule that is capable of combining with hydrogen ions and therefore lowers the hydrogen ion concentration of a solution.
   a. true
   b. false

   a

3. The pH of a solution is defined as
   a. the concentration of OH^- ions expressed as a logarithm.
   b. the negative logarithm of the hydrogen ion concentration.
   c. the number of acids in solution.
   d. the number of bases in solution.
   b

4. The volatile carbonic acid is produced due to the
   a. production of carbon dioxide resulting from oxidation of foodstuffs.
   b. production of hydrogen ions from lactic acid.
   c. release of bases from the liver during exercise.
   d. None of the above arc correct.
   a

5. The most common and strongest organic acid produced in skeletal muscle during heavy exercise is
   a. phosphoric acid.
   b. lactic acid.
   c. acetoacetic acid.
   d. None of the above are correct.
   b

6. An increase in the hydrogen ion concentration in contracting skeletal muscle can impair performance by hydrogen ions competing with calcium ions for binding sites on troponin.
   a. true
   b. false
   a

7. The first line of defense in protecting against pH change in contracting skeletal muscle is buffers located in the
   a. extracellular fluid.
   b. blood.
   c. cell.
   d. liver.
   c

8. The blood contains three principal buffer systems:
   a. proteins, hemoglobin, and bicarbonate.
   b. proteins, myoglobin, and bicarbonate.
   c. hemoglobin, myoglobin, and proteins.
   d. hemoglobin, proteins, and carbonic anhydrase.
   a

9. The bicarbonate buffer system is considered to be one of the most important blood buffer systems during exercise.
   a. true
   b. false
   a

10. The respiratory system works in the regulation of acid-base balance by lowering the blood tension of
    a. O_2
    b. CO_2
    c. HCO_3
    d. H_2CO_3
    b

11. One of the principal means by which the kidneys regulate acid-base balance is by increasing or decreasing the bicarbonate concentration of the blood.
    a. true
    b. false
    a

12. The principal buffer against acidosis during exercise is intracellular phosphate groups.
    a. true
    b. false
    b

13. Muscle pH is generally
    a. 0.4–0.6 pH units lower than blood pH.
    b. 0.4–0.6 pH units higher than blood pH.
    c. equal to blood pH.
    d. None of the above are correct.
    a

14. Sodium bicarbonate has been ingested by athletes in an attempt to
    a. improve performance by increasing blood buffering capacity.
    b. improve performance by decreasing muscle lactate production.
    c. improve performance by stimulating pulmonary ventilation to increase oxygen transport.
    d. Both (a) and (b) are correct.
    a

15. The amount of lactic acid produced during exercise is dependent on
    a. the exercise intensity.
    b. the amount of muscle mass involved.
    c. the duration of exercise.
    d. All of the above are correct.
    d

16. The kidneys do not play an important role in the regulation of acid-base balance during acute exercise.
    a. true
    b. false
    a

17. Intracellular proteins contribute approximately _____ of the muscle cell's buffering capacity.
    a. 10%
    b. 20%
    c. 40%
    d. 60%
    d

18. Muscle bicarbonate contributes approximately _____ of the cell's buffering capacity.
    a. 10%
    b. 20–30%
    c. 60%
    d. None of the above are correct.
    b

Suggested Lab Experiences

Several laboratory exercises could be employed to improve students' understanding of the acid-base regulation during exercise. Suggested lab experiences include:

1. *Measurement of pH during incremental exercise.* The objective of this laboratory experience is to demonstrate the changes in blood lactate concentration, pH, and bicarbonate concentration during incremental exercise. A volunteer subject could perform a graded exercise test with blood samples obtained via venipuncture or indwelling catheter at selected work rates for measurement of blood pH, HCO_3^-, and lactate concentrations.

2. *In vitro demonstration of buffering principles.* The objective of this lab experience is to demonstrate the effect of varying amounts of a buffer (e.g., sodium bicarbonate) on the resulting change in pH when lactic acid is added to a solution. For example, a lactic acid solution could be added to test tubes containing saline with varying bicarbonate concentrations (e.g., 15, 24, and 30mEq/l). Measurement of the resulting pH would demonstrate the effects of bicarbonate as a blood buffer.

Chapter 12 Temperature Regulation

Lecture Outline

Key Points	*Subpoints*	*Examples*
Importance of temperature regulation	1. Animals who maintain a rather constant body temperature are called homeotherms 2. Large increases in body temperature (i.e., from 37°C to 45°C) result in protein destruction and may result in death	Humans, dogs, horses
Overview of heat balance during exercise	1. Goal of temperature regulation is to prevent overheating and overcooling during exercise 2. During exercise, body temperature is regulated by making adjustments in the amount of heat that is lost 3. Body temperature varies a great deal (i.e., from core to skin)	Increased sweat rate

Key Points	*Subpoints*	*Examples*
Temperature measurement during exercise	1. Core temperature can be measured via rectal probes, tympanic measurement, or esophageal measurement 2. Skin temperature is usually measured at a series of sites and a weighted average computed	
Heat loss	1. The hypothalamus serves as the temperature control center—works like a thermostat 2. Heat production occurs during exercise due to muscular efficiency being only 20%–25%—the remaining energy loss is given off as heat	
	3. Heat loss occurs via four processes: (a) radiation; (b) conduction; (c) convection; and (d) evaporation	Evaporation is the most important means of heat loss during exercise; however, high %RH greatly reduces the rate of evaporation
	4. Vapor pressure gradient between the skin and environment dictates the rate of evaporation	
	5. The body can lose 0.58 kcal of heat for each ml of water that evaporates	Evaporation of 250 ml sweat = 160 kcal heat loss ($0.58 \times 250 = 160$)
The body's thermostat	1. Principal control center is the hypothalamus 2. Anterior hypothalamus is principally responsible for regulation of heat loss	

Key Points	*Subpoints*	*Examples*
	3. The posterior hypothalamus is responsible for reacting to a decrease in body temperature	
	4. Input to the hypothalamus comes from thermal receptors located in the skin and core	
	5. The hypothalamic "set point" refers to a reference temperature that the temperature control center tries to preserve by regulation of heat loss	A fever may result from an alteration in the "set point" due to pyrogens
Thermal events during exercise	1. Heat production by contracting skeletal muscles during exercise is directly proportional to the exercise intensity	i.e., ~ 5 kcal/liter O_2 consumption
	2. During exercise in a cool/dry environment, core temperature is directly proportional to the metabolic rate	
	3. Exercise in a hot/humid environment results in a greater increase in core temperature when compared to work in a cool environment due to the compromised ability to lose heat via evaporation	Heat injury may occur during prolonged work in a hot/humid environment if core temperature exceeds 41°C–42°C

Key Points	*Subpoints*	*Examples*
	4. Heat injury can be prevented by avoiding long periods of heat exposure, drinking adequate liquids during exercise, and exposing maximum surface for evaporation	Heat illness symptoms include nausea, dizziness, and a reduction in sweat rate
Heat acclimatization	1. Heat acclimatization is a series of physiological adjustments designed to minimize disturbances in homeostasis due to heat stress	
	2. The primary adjustments that occur due to heat acclimatization are: (a) earlier onset of sweating; (b) higher sweat rate; (c) reduced salt in sweat; (d) increased plasma volume; and (e) reduced skin blood flow	Acclimatization results in a 10%–12% increase in plasma proteins
Exercise in a cold environment	1. Exercise in a cold environment greatly reduces the chance of heat injury	
	2. In general, the combination of metabolic heat production and warm clothing prevents the development of hypothermia	Swimming in cold water may present a potential problem for hypothermia
	3. Individuals with a high percentage of fat have an advantage over lean individuals in cold tolerance	

Key Points	*Subpoints*	*Examples*
Cold acclimatization	Cold acclimatization results in three principal physiological adaptations: (a) reduction in skin temperature at which shivering begins—probably due to nonshivering thermogenesis; (b) improved intermittent peripheral vasodilation resulting in a higher hand temperature; and (c) improved ability to sleep in a cold environment	Mountain climbers

Exam Questions

1. The regulation of body temperature is critical because cellular structures and metabolic pathways are affected by temperature.
   a. true
   b. false
   a

2. During exercise, body temperature is regulated by making adjustments in the amount of heat that is lost.
   a. true
   b. false
   a

3. Within the body, temperature
   a. varies a great deal with the highest temperatures being maintained in the core.
   b. varies a great deal with the highest temperatures being at the skin.
   c. does not vary from organ to organ.
   d. None of the above are correct.
   a

4. The body's thermostat is located in the
   a. cerebellum.
   b. brain stem.
   c. hypothalamus.
   d. thalamus.
   c

5. The principal means of heat loss during running in a cool environment (20° C/low humidity) is via
   a. radiation.
   b. conduction.
   c. evaporation.
   d. convection.
   c

6. The transfer of heat from the body into molecules of cooler objects in contact with its surface is called
   a. radiation.
   b. conduction.
   c. convection.
   d. None of the above are correct.
   b

7. In general, at high environmental temperatures, the most important variable determining heat loss by evaporation is
   a. the ambient relative humidity.
   b. the amount of heat loss due to radiation.
   c. the amount of heat loss due to conduction.
   d. None of the above are correct.

   a

8. The posterior hypothalamus is responsible for reacting to a decrease in body temperature.
   a. true
   b. false

   a

9. Thermal receptors are located
   a. only within the skin.
   b. only in the spinal cord.
   c. within the skin, hypothalamus, and spinal cord.
   d. only within the hypothalamus.

   c

10. An increase in deep body temperature results in
    a. a decrease in skin blood flow.
    b. an increase in skin blood flow.
    c. a decrease in brain blood flow.
    d. None of the above are correct.

    b

11. In general, during exercise in a thermoneutral environment, the increase in core temperature is directly related to the exercise intensity.
    a. true
    b. false

    a

12. The primary adaptations that occur during heat acclimatization are
    a. a decreased plasma volume, earlier onset of sweating, and higher sweat rate.
    b. an increased plasma volume, earlier onset of sweating, and a higher seat rate.
    c. an increased plasma volume and lower sweat rate.
    d. None of the above are correct.

    b

13. Hypothermia is defined as
    a. a large decrease in skin temperature.
    b. a large decrease in core (body) temperature.
    c. a large increase in core temperature.
    d. None of the above are correct.

    b

14. Individuals with a high percentage of body fat have an advantage over lean individuals in tolerance to cold.
    a. true
    b. false

    a

15. Cold acclimatization results in an improved ability to sleep in a cold environment.
    a. true
    b. false

    a

16. Heat acclimatization occurs generally within
    a. two to three days.
    b. three to five days.
    c. seven to twelve days.
    d. fifteen to thirty days.

    c

17. Cold adaptation results in a reduction in the mean skin temperature at which shivering begins.
    a. true
    b. false
    a

18. A high percentage of body fat results in an increased ability to loose body heat during exercise.
    a. true
    b. false
    b

19. In response to a decrease in body temperature the _____ initiates the release of norepinephrine, which increases the rate of cellular metabolism.
    a. cerebrum
    b. posterior hypothalamus
    c. anterior hypothalamus
    d. medial hypothalamus
    b

20. Evaporation of one liter of sweat would result in the loss of _____ kcal of heat.
    a. 540
    b. 580
    c. 100
    d. 500
    b

Suggested Lab Experiences

Several laboratory exercises could be employed to improve students' understanding of temperature regulation during exercise. Suggested lab experiences include:

1. *Measurement of core and skin temperature during prolonged exercise.* The objective of this laboratory experience is to demonstrate the changes in core temperature, heart rate, and skin temperature that occur across time during constant load exercise (either cycle or treadmill). This experiment could be performed in a cool/dry environment or in a hot/humid environment.
2. *Calculation of heat production and elimination.* The objective of this lab is to estimate the amount of heat production during exercise and to estimate the amount of evaporation necessary to explain the resultant increase in body temperature.

Chapter 13 The Physiology of Training: Effect on $\dot{V}O_2$ max, Performance, Homeostasis, and Strength

Lecture Outline

Key Points	*Subpoints*	*Examples*
Exercise: a challenge to homeostasis	Physiological control systems must respond to maintain equilibrium during exercise	Body temperature
Principles of training	1. Overload	Muscle adaptations with weight training
	2. Specificity	Hypertrophy vs. mitochondria changes
$\dot{V}O_2$ max	1. Normal values	Table of values
	2. Changes with training	Figure showing changes relative to pretraining $\dot{V}O_2$ max
	3. Relationship of $\dot{V}O_2$ max to cardiac output and oxygen extraction	Show importance of stroke volume in this relationship
Factors affecting stroke volume	1. End diastolic volume	Increase in ventricular volume
	2. Contractility	Ejection fraction is high in untrained individuals
	3. Afterload	Less resistance offered by trained muscles in maximal exercise after training

Key Points	*Subpoints*	*Examples*
Factors affecting the a-$\overline{v}O_2$ difference	1. Capillary density	Increased number of capillaries per fiber after training
	2. Mitochondria number	Increased number after training
Effect of capillary density and mitochondria number on the oxygen deficit	$\dot{V}O_2$ reaches steady state faster	Show figure of change in oxygen deficit with training
Effect of capillary density and mitochondria number on sparing of blood glucose	1. More fat oxidation	Increased mitochondria allows increased FFA uptake and oxidation
	2. Less inhibition of FFA mobilization	Less lactate formation after training
Effect of training on blood pH	1. Less lactate formation	Decreased blood lactate after training
	2. Increased lactate uptake by liver and muscle after training	Higher blood flow to liver; shift in LDH in muscle
Central command vs. peripheral feedback as controllers of heart rate and ventilation responses during submaximal exercise	1. Lower physiological responses related to trained state of the active muscles	Heart rate lower in exercise involving trained muscles compared to using untrained muscles
	2. Fewer motor units needed to provide required tension after training	Trained muscle can provide greater power aerobically after training, and is more resistant to fatigue
Development of muscular strength	1. Neural mechanisms	Learning to recruit prime movers
	2. Hypertrophy	Increased cross-sectional area

Exam Questions

1. A cross-sectional study of the effect of endurance training would follow the same group of individuals over time.
   a. true
   b. false
   b

2. The average $\dot{V}O_2$ max value for the young male sedentary population is
   a. 35 ml • kg^{-1} - min^{-1}.
   b. 45 ml • kg^{-1} - min^{-1}.
   c. 55 ml • kg^{-1} - min^{-1}.
   d. 65 ml • kg^{-1} - min^{-1}.
   b

3. The variation in $\dot{V}O_2$ max among the various populations is due entirely to differences in the quantity and quality of training.
   a. true
   b. false
   b

4. The cardiovascular variable responsible for the large variation in $\dot{V}O_2$ max in the normal population is maximal
   a. heart rate.
   b. stroke volume.
   c. arteriovenous O_2 difference.
   b

5. Following training, if the increase in maximal cardiac output is balanced with a decrease in resistance, the mean arterial blood pressure will
   a. increase.
   b. decrease.
   c. remain the same.
   c

6. In a "two-legged" maximal cycle ergometer test, if each leg were to vasodilate to the extent experienced in a one-legged $\dot{V}O_2$ max test, mean arterial blood pressure would fall below normal levels.
   a. true
   b. false
   a

7. Following an endurance training program, there is usually a smaller oxygen deficit when the subject does the same work task. This is due to
   a. an increased cardiac output.
   b. increases in the number of mitochondria and capillaries.
   c. an increased heart rate.
   d. Both (b) and (c) are correct.
   b

8. The capacity of the trained muscle to use fatty acids as a fuel results in
   a. reduction in lactate formation.
   b. sparing of muscle glycogen.
   c. sparing of blood glucose.
   d. All of the above are correct.
   d

9. The change in lactate dehydrogenase in muscle with endurance training favors the formation of lactate.
   a. true
   b. false
   b

10. Lactate removal is greater following an endurance training program because blood flow to muscle is decreased and liver blood flow is increased at the same work rate.
    a. true
    b. false
    a

11. The changes in the heart rate and ventilatory responses to a fixed submaximal work rate are lower after an endurance training program. These changes are due primarily to
    a. changes in the lung and heart.
    b. changes in the active skeletal muscles.
    b

12. In the first 10 weeks of a resistance training program, the gains in strength are due, primarily, to
    a. neural adaptations.
    b. hypertrophy.
    a

Chapter 14 Factors Limiting Health and Fitness

Lecture Outline

Key Points	*Subpoints*	*Examples*
Causes of death in the United States	Infectious diseases vs. degenerative diseases	Figure showing changes during the twentieth century
Categories of risk factors	1. Genetic risk factors	Gender, race, age
	2. Environmental risk factors	Air and water quality; income and housing
	3. Behavioral risk factors	Smoking, inactivity, alcohol intake
Health risk appraisals	Predictors of disease	Smoking, elevated cholesterol, high blood pressure
Risk factors for coronary heart disease	1. Primary	Smoking, hypertension, inactivity, and elevated serum cholesterol
	2. Secondary	Stress, diabetes, obesity
Healthy People 2000	1. Physical activity	Increase physical activity of proper intensity, frequency, and duration
	2. Nutrition	Increase iron intake in women; decrease fat and salt intake

Exam Questions

1. The major causes of death in the United States are infectious diseases.
   a. true
   b. false
   b

2. In the wellness model, who has primary responsibility for taking care of one's heath?
   a. the physician
   b. each individual
   c. public health service
   d. schools
   b

3. The risk factors associated with degenerative diseases and death that are most susceptible to change include
   a. age.
   b. inactivity.
   c. water pollution.
   d. Both (b) and (c) are correct.
   d

4. A health risk appraisal
   a. is a substitute for a physical exam.
   b. predicts future disease with absolute accuracy.
   c. assesses the potential risk of disease based on current status.
   d. should be used with diseased populations.
   c

5. A secondary risk factor is one that increases the risk of coronary heart disease when no other risk factors are present.
   a. true
   b. false
   b

Suggested Lab Experiences

1. Have each student fill out an HRA and discuss the results relative to the categories selected.
2. If a computer-based HRA is available, have each student answer the questions. When each has a copy of the summary report, discuss the results.
3. Read the *Healthy People 2000* objectives to the class to focus their attention on the need to change certain behaviors in order to improve health status.

Chapter 15 Work Tests to Evaluate Cardiorespiratory Fitness

Lecture Outline

Key Points	*Subpoints*	*Examples*
Preliminary steps leading to the evaluation of cardiorespiratory fitness	1. Consent form	
	2. Health history	PAR-Q
	3. Decision tree	See text
Field tests to evaluate cardiorespiratory fitness	1. Maximal run tests	Cooper's 1.5-mile run
	2. Walk test	Use mile time and heart rate response in one-mile walk
	3. Canadian home fitness test	Step test
Graded Exercise Test (GXT)	1. Measurements	Heart rate, blood pressure RPE, ECG, $\dot{V}O_2$ max
	2. Estimation of $\dot{V}O_2$ max	Use last work rate achieved in maximal test; extrapolate HR response from submaximal work rates
	3. Termination criteria	Signs, symptoms, ECG changes, HR and BP responses
	4. Protocols	Treadmill—walk vs. run; cycle ergometer—YMCA or Åstrand-Ryhming nomogram; step test

Exam Questions

1. If a thirty-year-old man checked a "yes" response in the PAR-Q, what should he do prior to taking an exercise test?
   a. nothing; he can take the test
   b. contact his physician for permission to take the test
   c. have a complete physical exam
   d. check into a hospital immediately
   b

2. The basis of the Cooper field test for estimating $\dot{V}O_2$ max is
   a. maximal heart rate is achieved during the test.
   b. the average running speed is below the anaerobic threshold.
   c. the average running speed is dependent on oxygen uptake.
   d. maximal running speed is attained.
   c

3. A sign of ischemia measured on an ECG during a graded exercise test is
   a. a large P wave.
   b. an increase in the width of a QRS complex.
   c. a depression of the ST segment.
   d. a disappearance of the T wave.
   c

4. Which of the following is not a criterion for having achieved $\dot{V}O_2$ max during a graded exercise test?
   a. leveling off of the $\dot{V}O_2$ with increasing work rate
   b. achieving 85% of maximal heart rate
   c. a blood lactate level of 10 mmoles • liter^{-1}
   d. respiratory exchange ratio of 1.20
   b

5. The highest $\dot{V}O_2$ max value is usually measured during a
   a. cycle ergometer test.
   b. graded treadmill walk test to exhaustion.
   c. graded treadmill run test to exhaustion.
   d. arm ergometer test.
   c

6. Using a graded exercise test in which the work rate increments are large and the duration of each stage is short will result in an underestimation of $\dot{V}O_2$ max based on the last work load achieved.
   a. true
   b. false
   b

7. $\dot{V}O_2$ max is estimated for a forty-year-old man by drawing a line through the heart rate values measured during a submaximal graded exercise test and extrapolating to the age-adjusted maximal heart rate. This estimate
   a. may be low because the age-adjusted maximal heart rate may actually be 165 beats • min^{-1}.
   b. may be high because the age-adjusted maximal heart rate may actually be 165 beats • min^{-1}.
   c. is always accurate because the age-adjusted maximal heart rate is accurate.
   d. None of the above are correct.
   b

8. For which of the following reasons would you stop a graded exercise test?
   a. heart rate increases with increasing work rate
   b. diastolic blood pressure remains the same with increasing work rate
   c. systolic blood pressure remains the same with increasing work rate
   d. ST segment is not depressed with increasing work rate

   c

9. A single GXT protocol is suitable for all populations.
   a. true
   b. false

   b

10. The YMCA uses a flowchart to plot the course of a GXT. Which of the following statements is true relative to that test?
    a. A small increase in heart rate from stage one to stage two of the GXT would result in a large change in the work rate for the next stage of the test.
    b. It is better to move through the stages quickly so the test does not last too long.
    c. The test for the less fit individual would tend to have large increases in the work rate from one stage to the next.

    a

Suggested Lab Experiences

1. Have each student fill out the PAR-Q and, based on the responses, follow the directions indicated on the form.
2. Have each student walk as fast as possible over a one-mile course and measure:
   a. the time of the walk
   b. a ten-second heart rate, initiated within five seconds of the end of the run. Then, with these numbers have them calculate $\dot{V}O_2$ max using the equation in the text.
3. Have each student complete a 1.5-mile run (after warming up and stretching) on a measured track. They should maintain a steady pace and not walk. Calculate the average running speed by dividing the metric equivalent of 1.5 miles (2,414 meters) by the time measured in minutes and tenths of minutes (calculated by dividing the number of seconds by 60). This average running speed is then used in the equation in the text to calculate $\dot{V}O_2$ max from running speed.
4. Do a submaximal graded exercise test on a cycle, step, or treadmill to 85% of the student's maximal heart rate, and extrapolate to the age-adjusted estimate of maximal heart rate to estimate $\dot{V}O_2$ max. Various GXT protocols are identified in the text.

Chapter 16 Training for Health and Fitness

Lecture Outline

Key Points	*Subpoints*	*Examples*
The changing perception of inactivity as a risk factor	Moderate activity is sufficient to reduce CHD risk	Center for Disease Control; Paffenbarger alumni study
Exercise and the risk of cardiac arrest	Compare risk during physical activity with the overall risk	Risk is higher during activity, but lower overall
Health benefits of physical activity go beyond the increase in $\dot{V}O_2$ max	Risk factors are altered	Serum cholesterol and fibrinolysis activity are favorably altered with physical activity
Screening and progression are important when initiating an exercise program	1. Health history 2. Do too little rather than too much 3. Warm-up and cool down	PAR-Q Complete walk program before starting jog program Begin and end exercise session with light activity and stretching
Exercise prescription	1. Optimum intensity 2. Optimum frequency 3. Optimum duration	60%–80% $\dot{V}O_2$ max; 70%–85% HR max, 60%–80% heart rate range Three to four days per week Sufficient to expend 200–300 kcal
Target heart rate controls for environmental conditions	Heat, altitude, and pollution can elevate the HR during exercise	Monitor heart rate and reduce exercise intensity when environmental factors increase heart rate

Key Points	*Subpoints*	*Examples*
Strength training	Needed for activities of daily living, and to maintain lean body mass	Do 10 to 12 reps of 8 to 10 different exercises at least twice a week

Exam Questions

1. Based on the most recent evidence, which of the following is a secondary risk factor for heart disease?
   a. inactivity
   b. high serum cholesterol
   c. high blood pressure
   d. None of the above are correct.
   d

2. Compared to the resting state, the risk of a cardiac arrest during vigorous exercise for the habitually active person is
   a. higher.
   b. lower.
   c. the same.
   d. None of the above are correct.
   a

3. The risk of injuries and cardiovascular problems associated with increasing levels of physical activity
   a. increases linearly with level of activity.
   b. is low at low-to-moderate levels of physical activity.
   c. is low for all levels of physical activity.
   d. is high for all levels of physical activity.
   b

4. The increase in $\dot{V}O_2$ max due to vigorous activity is the only reason that exercise is associated with a lower risk of heart disease.
   a. true
   b. false
   b

5. The optimum range of intensity of physical activity associated with gains in $\dot{V}O_2$ max is about
   a. 30%–65% $\dot{V}O_2$ max.
   b. 40%–75% $\dot{V}O_2$ max.
   c. 50%–85% $\dot{V}O_2$ max.
   d. 60%–95% $\dot{V}O_2$ max.
   c

6. The optimum number of times per week to exercise to achieve cardiorespiratory fitness goals is
   a. one to two.
   b. three to four.
   c. five to six.
   d. seven.
   b

7. Given: 50-year-old man with a resting heart rate of 70 beats • min^{-1}. What is the target heart rate range as determined by the heart rate reserve method?
   a. 130–150 beats • min^{-1}
   b. 102–144 beats • min^{-1}
   c. 120–140 beats • min^{-1}
   d. 140–155 beats • min^{-1}
   a

8. The optimal training intensity using Borg's original scale is
   a. 6–8.
   b. 8–10.
   c. 10–12.
   d. 12–14.
   d

9. A 30-year-old woman achieves target heart rate on a cool day by jogging at 6 mph. If she were to exercise at altitude or on a very hot day she would have to
   a. maintain the speed of her run to achieve her target heart rate.
   b. decrease the speed of her run to achieve her target heart rate.
   c. increase the speed of her run to achieve her target heart rate.
   b

Suggested Lab Experiences

1. Given the following case study, have each student identify the risk factors, calculate a target heart rate, and recommend an appropriate exercise program.

   Subject is 55-year-old sedentary black male, an executive at a nearby computer corporation. His job requires him to be out of town two to three days per week, and he generally feels an inability to get everything done. He smokes 1.5 packs of cigarettes a day. His mother died of a stroke at the age of 68 and his father died of a heart attack at the age of 70. Physical characteristics: Height = 70 inches, weight = 188 lbs., and has 23% body fat. His resting blood pressure is 130/85 and his resting pulse rate is 76. Blood chemistry values were: total cholesterol = 300 mg/dl; HDL cholesterol = 35/mgdl; glucose = 100 md/dl; triglycerides = 190 mg/dl. The results of a graded exercise test follow:

   Speed 3 mph

Grade	*Mets*	*Heart Rate*	*Blood Pressure*	*RPE*	*Comments*
2.5%	4.3	110	105/84	9	EKG-ok
5.0%	5.4	124	160/84	11	EKG-ok
7.5%	6.4	138	175/86	13	EKG-ok
10%	7.4	156	190/84	15	EKG-ok
12.5%	8.5	180	200/86	18	Fatigue

1. List the primary and secondary risk factors.
2. Would you enroll this person in an exercise program without further referral? Why?
3. What might you suggest to this individual?
4. What is your reaction to the results of his stress test?
5. Calculate a THR range for this person.
6. Recommend an exercise program for this person, including the types of activities, duration, frequency, and so on.

Chapter 17 Exercise for Special Populations

Lecture Outline

Key Points	*Subpoints*	*Examples*
Diabetics and exercise	1. Types	Type I: Insulin-dependent Type II: Adult onset or non-insulin dependent
	2. Too much or too little insulin	Insulin shock or diabetic coma
	3. Control blood glucose	Vary diet and insulin depending on exercise intensity and duration and level of blood glucose prior to exercise
Asthmatics and exercise	1. Asthma attack	Bronchoconstriction, swelling of mucosal cells, and increased secretions
	2. Prevention of exercise-induced attack	Use drugs before and during exercise; use long warm-up; prevent drying of the airway
Chronic obstructive pulmonary disease and exercise	1. Long-term lung disease	Bronchitis, emphysema, and bronchial asthma
	2. Rehabilitation and self-care	Medical care and services of social workers, clergy, psychologists, etc., needed
Hypertension	1. Dietary intervention	Reduce salt and caloric intake
	2. Exercise	Do light exercise for 30 to 60 minutes, 3 to 4 times per week

Key Points	*Subpoints*	*Examples*
Exercise for the cardiac patient	1. Variety of patients	Angina, myocardial infarction, bypass surgery, and angioplasty
	2. Testing	Monitor 12-lead ECG
	3. Exercise program	Patients are monitored for HR/ECG and supervised by medical personnel
Exercise for the elderly	1. Classification	Young old, old old, and athletic old
	2. Exercise program varies with classification	Maintains cardiovascular fitness and bone integrity
Exercise and pregnancy	1. Physician supervised	Follow physician's directions
	2. Conservative exercise prescription	Less than 140 b/min; short duration; no Valsalva maneuvers; no supine exercise after the fourth month

Exam Questions

1. The majority of diabetics are classified as Type II diabetics.
   a. true
   b. false
   a

2. If a Type I diabetic engages in exercise while the blood glucose concentration is too high, the exercise will cause the blood glucose concentration to increase.
   a. rue
   b. false
   a

3. Insulin shock is a condition in which the diabetic is
   a. hyperglycemic.
   b. hypoglycemic.
   c. ketotic.
   d. All of the above are correct.
   b

4. A condition that is regarded as a cause of Type II diabetes is
   a. obesity.
   b. too much sugar in the diet.
   c. a high-protein diet.
   d. extremely low body weight.
   a

5. An asthma attack that is brought on by exercise can be prevented by
   a. taking proper medication prior to exercise.
   b. exercising at a very high intensity.
   c. breathing air that has been cooled and dried.
   d. All of the above are correct.

   a

6. Patients with COPD have a lower tolerance for exercise than do cardiac patients.
   a. true
   b. false

   a

7. A cardiac patient who has had angioplasty to correct a problem has had
   a. veins sutured to the coronary arteries.
   b. a pacemaker installed in the right atrium.
   c. the lumen of a coronary artery increased.
   d. a heart attack.

   c

8. The "athletic old" group of the elderly
   a. is severely limited in the activities they can do.
   b. can do most of the activities that middle-aged sedentary people do.
   c. need special supervision, similar to that of Phase I cardiac programs.
   d. should not engage in exercise.

   b

9. Exercise is not recommended for the pregnant woman because it puts an additional strain on the fetus.
   a. true
   b. false

   b

Suggested Lab Experiences

1. Have each member of the class visit an exercise program for one of the groups discussed in this chapter, and write a brief report of the findings. Hold a class discussion about the results when all the reports are in.

Chapter 18 Body Composition and Nutrition for Health

Lecture Outline

Key Points	*Subpoints*	*Examples*
U.S. Dietary Goals and Dietary Guidelines for Americans	Change diet for health	Increase intake of complex carbohydrates; decrease fat and salt intake
Standards for nutrition	RDA and the U.S. RDA	Optimal quantity of vitamins, minerals, and protein needed for health
Vitamins	1. Water-soluble	B vitamins, vitamin C, niacin, folic acid, pantothenic acid, and biotin
	2. Fat-soluble	Vitamins A, D, E, and K
Minerals	1. Major minerals	Calcium, phosphorus, potassium, sulfur, sodium, chloride, and magnesium
	2. Trace elements	Iron, zinc, copper, iodine, manganese, selenium, molybdenum, cobalt, arsenic, nickel, fluoride, and vanadium
Optimum amount of carbohydrate and fat for health	1. Increase complex carbohydrates and decrease sugars	Increase intake of cereals, whole-grain breads, and fruits; decrease intake of soft drinks, jams, cakes, and cookies
	2. Decrease fat intake	Choose lean meats; eat more fish and poultry; trim fat off meat; broil rather than fry

Key Points	*Subpoints*	*Examples*
Meal plans for healthy diets	1. Food Guide Pyramid	Includes meats, milk, breads, fruits, and vegetables
	2. Exchange System	Foods are classed by caloric content and percent of fat, protein, and carbohydrate
Body composition analysis	1. Techniques	Summarize those listed in text
	2. Two-component model of body composition	Fat mass and lean mass
	3. Underwater weighing	Principle; error in measurement; "standard"
	4. Skinfold technique	Sum of skinfold thicknesses is used to predict body density, using the underwater weighing as the standard
Body composition and health	Optimal fat percentage	10%–20% for males, and 15%–25% for females
Obesity	1. Hyperplasia vs. hypertrophy of fat cells	Growth in fat cell number; relation of fat mass to cell number
	2. Genetics vs. environment	Body fatness relationship of adoptees and parents; fatness of children compared to parents
RMR and weight loss	1. Small changes in resting metabolic rate can affect body fatness	Decrease of only 10 kcal per day could lead to a gain of one pound per year
	2. Low-calorie diets	RMR decreases
	3. Exercise	Exercise maintains the lean body mass, but probably does affect the metabolic rate of the lean body mass

Key Points	*Subpoints*	*Examples*
Exercise, appetite, and body composition	1. Proportional intake of calories to balance expenditure if doing moderate activity	Mayer's rat study
	2. Lack of proportional increase in appetite with exercise intervention	Suggests that a sudden increase in activity is not followed by an increase in appetite
	3. Lean mass increased or maintained with exercise	Exercise plus diet maintains more of the lean body mass than a diet-alone weight-loss program

Exam Questions

1. As recommended by the U.S. Dietary Goals, what percentage of calories in the American diet should come from carbohydrate?
   a. 35–40
   b. 45–50
   c. 55–60
   d. 65–70
   c

2. The U.S. RDA standards specify the amounts of each vitamin, mineral, and protein needed for optimal health.
   a. true
   b. false
   b

3. An excessive consumption of which of the following vitamins can lead to a toxicity?
   a. A
   b. thiamin
   c. riboflavin
   d. niacin
   a

4. Which of the following major minerals, when inadequate, can increase the chance of bone fractures in the elderly?
   a. sodium
   b. calcium
   c. chloride
   d. potassium
   b

5. Which of the following trace minerals is related to anemia?
   a. zinc
   b. iodine
   c. iron
   d. fluoride
   c

6. In an attempt to deal with some forms of hypertension, which of the following major minerals should be reduced in the diet of the average American?
   a. sodium
   b. calcium
   c. chloride
   d. potassium

   a

7. On a per gram basis, fats have more than twice as many calories as carbohydrates.
   a. true
   b. false

   a

8. A high level of which of the following type of serum cholesterol is related to a low risk of heart disease?
   a. total cholesterol
   b. HDL-cholesterol
   c. LDL-cholesterol

   b

9. The type of dietary fat that is linked to increased heart disease is contained in which of the following products?
   a. corn oil
   b. olive oil
   c. butter

   c

10. The Food Guide Pyramid includes the following groups:
    a. milk, meat, grains, and water.
    b. milk, meat, fruits, vegetables, and breads.
    c. meat, fruits/vegetables, grains, and water.
    d. None of the above are correct.

    b

11. The Exchange System focuses on which of the following food characteristics?
    a. calories
    b. percent of carbohydrate, fat, and protein
    c. nutrient density
    d. Both (a) and (b) are correct.

    d

12. The body composition method that uses an isotope of iodine to measure the density of bones is
    a. isotope dilution.
    b. photon absorptiometry.
    c. potassium-40.
    d. radiography.

    b

13. In the densitometry method of body composition analysis, the density of the body is compared to the density of
    a. fat.
    b. muscle.
    c. bone.
    d. water.

    d

14. Some of the error in estimating body fatness from body density measurements is related to variability in the density of
    a. the fat mass.
    b. the lean mass.
    c. water.

    b

15. If you did not correct the underwater weight for the air remaining in the lungs at the time of measurement, you would underestimate body fatness.
    a. true
    b. false

    b

16. The optimal body fatness range for males is
    a. 5%–10%.
    b. 10%–15%.
    c. 10%–20%.
    d. 15%–25%.
    c

17. The optimal body fatness range for females is
    a. 5%–10%.
    b. 10%–15%.
    c. 10%–20%.
    d. 15%–25%.
    d

18. The type of obesity that is due to an increase in the fat cell number is called hypertrophic obesity.
    a. true
    b. false
    b

19. On the basis of studies of adults over their lifespan, the gin is weight that occurs with age is due to an increase in caloric intake.
    a. true
    b. false
    b

20. Individuals who cut their normal caloric intake in half experience a reduction in resting metabolic rate.
    a. true
    b. false
    a

21. The energy requirement for walking one mile is the same as that for jogging one mile.
    a. true
    b. false
    b

Suggested Lab Experiences

1. Have each student complete a three-day food record and have them determine:
    a. how well they meet the guidelines for the basic Food Guide Pyramid
    b. how many calories they consumed each day
    c. what percentage of calories comes from carbohydrates, fats, and protein.
2. Measure body fatness by the skinfold technique and discuss the values measured in the class with those associated with good health.
3. Measure the resting metabolic rate on each student and discuss the variation of this measure with regard to the ease or difficulty of staying in energy balance.

Chapter 19 Factors Affecting Performance

Lecture Outline

Key Points	*Subpoints*	*Examples*
Overview of factors affecting performance	1. Skill	Sport-specific skills such as throwing, dribbling etc.
	2. Energy	Aerobic and anaerobic
	3. Nutrition	Carbohydrates and water
	4. Environment	Heat and altitude
	5. Motivation	Desire to win
	6. Strength and power	Weight lifting, shot putting, javelin throwing etc.
Central nervous system as the site of fatigue	1. Evidence against	Voluntary vs. electrically induced contractions
	2. Evidence for	A "shout" can increase "maximal" strength; use of a diversion increases work output
Periphery as the site of fatigue	1. Neuromuscular junction	Evidence suggests this is not the site of fatigue
	2. Sarcolemma and T-tubule	Rapid stimulation of a muscle may be associated with a slower rate of conduction
	3. Mechanical factors	Elevated H^+ concentration in muscle may interfere with the ability of troponin to bind Ca^{++}
	4. Energetics	Muscle fibers relying on anaerobic sources of energy fatigue quickly

Key Points	*Subpoints*	*Examples*
Factors limiting maximal performances lasting < 10 seconds	1. Muscle fiber type	Fast-twitch fibers will generate more power
	2. Energy sources	Creatine phosphate store with anaerobic glycolysis
	3. Skill	Practice
Factors limiting maximal performances of 10 to 180 seconds	1. Muscle fiber type	Fast-twitch fibers have an advantage
	2. Energy sources	Creatine phosphate, with glycolysis playing a more important role; aerobic production of ATP becoming important
Factors limiting maximal performances of 3 to 20 minutes	1. Maximal oxygen uptake	Values range from as low as 40 ml • kg^{-1} • min^{-1} in young sedentary males to 80 ml • kg^{-1} • min^{-1} in elite distance runners
	2. Maximal stroke volume	Determined by genetics and training
	3. Arterial oxygen content	Determined by hemoglobin concentration, barometric pressure, and the fraction of inspired oxygen
	4. Mixed venous oxygen content	Determined by the fiber types and their mitochondrial contents
Factors limiting maximal performances of 21 to 60 minutes	1. High steady state $\dot{V}O_2$	Greater energy production to run at a higher speed
	2. Lactate threshold	Good estimate of the intensity that can be maintained in long runs
	3. Environmental factors	Heat load and altitude
	4. Running economy	Running speed is higher in more economical runner at same $\dot{V}O_2$

Key Points	*Subpoints*	*Examples*
Factors limiting maximal performances of one to four hours	1. High steady state $\dot{V}O_2$	Greater energy production to run at a higher speed
	2. Lactate threshold	Good estimate of the intensity that can be maintained in long runs
	3. Environmental factors	Heat load and altitude
	4. Nutritional factors	High-carbohydrate diet
	5. Running economy	Running speed is higher in more economical runner at same $\dot{V}O_2$

Exam Questions

1. A subject, with eyes closed, repeatedly contracts a muscle until fatigue occurs. When the eyes are opened, tension is restored. This experiment is a demonstration of fatigue being related to which of the following sites?
   a. muscle
   b. central nervous system
   c. mitochondria
   d. peripheral nervous system
   b

2. What by-product of heavy muscular exercise may actually interfere with the interaction of Ca^{++} and troponin?
   a. H^+
   b. creatine
   c. CO_2
   d. ketone bodies
   a

3. When the intensity of exercise exceeds 75% $\dot{V}O_2$ max, which of the following fibers is brought into play?
   a. Type I
   b. Type IIA
   c. Type IIB
   d. Type IIC
   c

4. In ultra short-term performances (less than 10 seconds), which of the following factors is the primary cause of fatigue?
   a. muscle glycogen depletion
   b. creatine phosphate depletion
   c. hypoglycemia
   d. depression of plasma FFA
   b

5. In short-term performances (10–180 seconds) which of the following factors is the primary cause of fatigue?
   a. muscle glycogen depletion
   b. depressed plasma FFA
   c. hypoglycemia
   d. H^+ accumulation

   d

6. In aerobic performances lasting three to twenty minutes, which of the following factors limits performance?
   a. $\dot{V}O_2$ max
   b. creatine phosphate depletion
   c. hypoglycemia
   d. depression of plasma FFA

   a

7. In running performances lasting 21 to 60 minutes, the only factor limiting performance is $\dot{V}O_2$ max.
   a. true
   b. false

   b

8. In running performances lasting one to four hours, which of the following factors may limit performance?
   a. $\dot{V}O_2$ max
   b. creatine phosphate depletion
   c. availability of carbohydrate
   d. depression of plasma FFA

   c

Chapter 20 Work Tests to Evaluate Performance

Lecture Outline

Key Points	*Subpoints*	*Examples*
Two principal approaches to assessment of physical performance	1. Field test 2. Lab assessments	12-minute run Measurement of $\dot{V}O_2$ max
Lab assessments of physical performance	Physiological testing: theory and ethics Direct measurement of $\dot{V}O_2$ max (a) Specificity of testing (b) Exercise test protocol (c) Peak $\dot{V}O_2$-arm work	Open-circuit spirometry Measurement of performance in paraplegic athletes
Use of lactate threshold to evaluate performance	1. Direct determination of lactate threshold during exercise 2. Prediction of lactate threshold via ventilatory alterations 3. Lactate threshold has been shown by several investigators to correlate closely with success in distance events	Progressive treadmill or cycle test Ventilatory threshold 10-kilometer run
Estimating success in distance running	1. Measurement of $\dot{V}O_2$ max 2. Measurement of the lactate threshold 3. Measurement of running economy	Correlates closely to distance running success in group of heterogenous athletes

Key Points	*Subpoints*	*Examples*
	4. Use of running economy and the lactate threshold can assist in prediction of the maximum speed that an athlete can maintain during an endurance race	10-kilometer run
Determination of anaerobic power	1. Margaria power test	F = 75 kg D = 2 meters T = 0.65s Power = 230.8 kgm/s
	2. Sargent's jump-and-reach test	
	3. Running power tests	40-yard dash used in football Stuart power test
	4. Cycling power tests (ultra-short)	Quebec 10-second test
	5. Tests of medium-term anaerobic power	Wingate test
Evaluation of muscular strength	1. 1-RM	Use of free weights to measure dynamic strength
	2. Dynamometry	Back lift
	3. Cable tensiometry	Technique used to measure isometric strength
	4. Computerized assessment of strength	Isokinetic measurement of strength offers several advantages over a 1 RM test in that information is supplied concerning the force generation over the entire range of movement

Exam Questions

1. Physical performance is a complex interaction of several factors, including maximal energy output, muscular strength, movement economy, and psychological factors.
   a. true
   b. false
   a

2. Measurement of $\dot{V}O_2$ max can be performed using either the arms or the legs.
   a. true
   b. false
   b

3. A $\dot{V}O_2$ max test can be considered of value if two of the following criteria are met:
   a. (1) R > 1.0; (2) HR max ±1 beat within predicted HR max; (3) blood lactate concentration > 6 mM.
   b. (1) R > 1.15; (2) HR max ± 10 beats within predicted HR max; (3) plateau in $\dot{V}O_2$ with increasing work rate.
   c. (1) R > 1.15; (2) ventilation > 100 liters/min; (3) plateau in blood lactate concentration with increasing work rate.
   d. None of the above are correct.
   b

4. Measurement of the highest $\dot{V}O_2$ obtained during an incremental arm ergometer test is often called
   a. $\dot{V}O_2$ max.
   b. peak $\dot{V}O_2$.
   c. maximal aerobic power.
   d. max $\dot{V}O_2$.
   b

5. Laboratory tests can be used to predict performance in distance running events by measurement of an athlete's lactate threshold, running economy, and $\dot{V}O_2$ max.
   a. true
   b. false
   a

6. The Wingate test provides an estimate of short-term (i.e., two-to-five second) anaerobic power output in athletes.
   a. true
   b. false
   b

7. Performance of a one-repetition maximum test to determine muscular strength is an example of a(n)
   a. isokinetic strength test.
   b. dynamic strength test.
   c. isometric strength test.
   d. None of the above are correct.
   b

8. The Sargent's jump and reach test is considered a good predictor of success in running a short dash.
   a. true
   b. false
   b

9. Which of the following factors are important to consider when designing a laboratory test to evaluate sport performance?
   a. tests should be both valid and reliable
   b. tests do not need to be sport specific
   c. tests should use both upper and lower body muscles
   d. Both (a) and (b) are correct.
   a

10. Measurement of the lactate threshold has been used to estimate
    a. maximal aerobic power.
    b. maximal steady-state running speed.
    c. maximal performance in events lasting less than 60 s.
    d. None of the above are correct.
    b

Suggested Lab Experiences

Several laboratory experiences could be employed to improve students' understanding of physical performance testing. Suggested lab experiences include:

1. *Measurement of $\dot{V}O_2$ max and peak $\dot{V}O_2$ during arm work.* The objective is to demonstrate the measurement of $\dot{V}O_2$ max and peak $\dot{V}O_2$ during incremental exercise. Measurement of pulmonary gas exchange can be managed with a computerized system or with Douglas bags, depending on availability.
2. *Measurement of running economy.* The objective is to measure running economy using several horizontal treadmill speeds. Data can then be graphed and used to predict the oxygen cost of running at various speeds.
3. *Prediction of running performance.* The objective of this lab experience is to use lactate threshold data and running economy measurements to predict performance in a 10-kilometer race. Data for the lactate threshold and running economy can be manufactured for class use or can result from actual laboratory measurements.
4. *Measurement of anaerobic power.* The objective of this lab experience is to measure anaerobic power using either or both the Margaria power test or the Wingate test.
5. *Measurement of a 1-RM test or isokinetic strength.* The objective is to demonstrate the use of a 1-RM test and/or a commercial isokinetic strength-testing device as a means of evaluating muscular strength. Advantages and disadvantages of each procedure can then be discussed.

Chapter 21 Training for Performance

Lecture Outline

Key Points	*Subpoints*	*Examples*
Training principles	1. Overall objective of sport conditioning is to improve performance by increasing the energy output during a particular movement	Generate more power when throwing the discus
	2. Important concepts to remember when designing conditioning programs include the principles of overload, specificity, and reversibility	
	3. Genetics and the initial fitness level of an individual play an important role in how an individual responds to a training program	Less fit individuals show a greater % improvement in response to training programs than better conditioned subjects
Components of a training session	1. Warm-up exercises are performed prior to a workout as a means of increasing muscle temperature, cardiac output, and muscle blood flow	
	2. Training sessions are designed to improve the energy systems employed in a particular sport	

Key Points	*Subpoints*	*Examples*
	3. A cool-down period allows pooled blood from the exercised skeletal muscles to return to the central circulation	
Training to improve $\dot{V}O_2$ max	1. Interval training	Repeated 400-meter dashes
	2. Long slow distance	10-mile slow run
	3. High-intensity continuous exercise	Hard 5-kilometer run
	4. Combined strength and endurance training programs	
Training for improved anaerobic power	1. Training to improve the ATP-CP system involves short-term, high-intensity efforts	Used in sports like football, weightlifting etc.
	2. Training to improve the glycolytic system involves high-intensity activities lasting 20 to 60 seconds	Useful for events like the 400-meter dash in track
Training to improve muscular strength	1. Isometric exercise	
	2. Isotonic exercise including variable resistance exercise	
	3. Isokinetic exercise	
	4. Progressive resistance exercise for increasing muscular strength was first introduced by Delorme and Watkins in 1948	Overload principle
	5. The ideal number of repetitions to achieve optimum strength improvement is generally believed to be between four to eight	Rest days between strength workouts appear to be important

Key Points	*Subpoints*	*Examples*
	6. Controversy exists around the question of whether training with free weights or various types of weight machines produces the greatest improvement in strength 7. Men and women appear to increase muscular strength in a similar fashion during short-term training periods. It is not clear if mean and women differ in strength gains over long-term weight training	
Delayed onset muscle soreness (DOMS)	1. DOMS is thought to occur due to tissue injury caused by excessive muscular force—occurs more frequently following eccentric exercise 2. The physiological explanation of DOMS is as follows: (a) excessive muscular force results in muscle damage; (b) Ca^{++} leaks out of muscle; (c) collection of Ca^{++} activates proteases, which degrade cellular proteins; (d) inflammatory process occurs; and (e) the accumulation of histamines, prostaglandins etc. irritates pain receptors	Soreness that occurs 24 to 48 hours post-exertion

Key Points	*Subpoints*	*Examples*
Training for improved flexibility	1. Static stretching	Thirty minutes of stretching two times per week will improve flexibility within five weeks
	2. Ballistic stretching	Static stretching is generally considered superior to ballistic stretching due to the reduction in injury probability
Year-round training for athletes	1. Off-season conditioning is useful in preventing fat weight gain, maintaining muscular strength, maintaining ligament and bone integrity, and maintaining a reasonable skill level in the athlete's specific sport	
	2. Preseason conditioning (8 to 12 weeks prior to season) is useful in increasing the maximum capacities of the predominant energy systems used in the sport	Common mistakes in training include overtraining, undertraining, using exercises and work rates that are not sport specific.
	3. In-season training is used to maintain the level of fitness achieved during the preseason conditioning period	

Exam Questions

1. A well-designed conditioning program allocates the appropriate amount of aerobic and anaerobic time to match the energy demand of the sport.
   a. true
   b. false
   a

2. The term *overload,* when used in conjunction with a sport conditioning program, means to
   a. overtrain or to exercise too much relative to the individual's capacity.
   b. stress the system above a level to which it's accustomed.
   c. injure or damage a muscle group.
   d. None of the above are correct.
   b

3. Evidence exists that men and women adapt differently to exercise training programs, which suggests that a different approach to physical conditioning must be taken for men and women.
   a. true
   b. false
   b

4. A genetic predisposition for athletic talent
   a. is not necessary for an individual to compete at a world-class level.
   b. has little impact on the individual's ultimate athletic potential.
   c. is essential if an individual is to compete at a world-class level.
   d. is important only in power events such as sprinting.
   c

5. A cool-down period following heavy exercise is probably very important in
   a. allowing the individual to reduce brain blood flow back to normal.
   b. returning "pooled" blood from the exercising skeletal muscle back to the central circulation.
   c. preventing heat stroke.
   d. None of the above are correct.
   b

6. In general, the longer the length or duration of the interval (i.e., interval training), the greater the contribution of anaerobic energy production during the interval.
   a. true
   b. false
   b

7. There is growing evidence that long, slow, distance training results in a greater improvement in $\dot{V}O_2$ max than high-intensity training.
   a. true
   b. false
   b

8. Intervals aimed at specific improvement of the ATP-CP system would generally last between
   a. 200–300 seconds.
   b. 5–10 seconds.
   c. 35–120 seconds.
   d. 30–90 seconds.
   b

9. Although the perfect training regimen for strength training is unknown, it is generally believed that the optimum number of repetitions per set is
   a. two to five.
   b. one to three.
   c. four to eight.
   d. ten to eighteen.

   c

10. Women involved in strength training programs do not gain strength as rapidly as men.
    a. true
    b. false

    b

11. Delayed onset of muscle soreness is thought to be due to
    a. lactic acid buildup in muscles.
    b. depletion of muscle glycogen.
    c. microscopic tears in the muscle resulting in calcium release from the SR.
    d. muscle cramps.

    c

12. Ballistic stretching is thought to be superior to static stretching due to a decreased chance of muscle injury.
    a. true
    b. false

    b

13. Off-season conditioning in athletes is useful in
    a. preventing excessive weight gain in the off-season.
    b. maintaining muscular strength.
    c. maintaining ligament and bone strength.
    d. All of the above are correct.

    d

Suggested Lab Experiences

1. Planning a preseason conditioning program for a selected sport. The objective of this written laboratory assignment is to provide the student an opportunity to develop a preseason training program for a sport(s) of their choice. The student should provide detailed weekly plans of conditioning activities as well as arguments to support their choices of drills.

Chapter 22 Training for Special Populations

Lecture Outline

Key Points	*Subpoints*	*Examples*
Competitive training for diabetics	1. It is generally considered safe for type I diabetics to engage in competitive training if the individual does not suffer from microvascular damage or neuropathy 2. The key to safe participation for the type I diabetic is to learn to avoid hypoglycemic episodes during training 3. Diabetics respond to training in a manner similar to nondiabetics	Distance running; swimming
Training for asthmatics	Asthmatics can participate in any sports activity if they are able to control or prevent exercise-induced bronchospasms	
Epilepsy and physical training	1. Epileptic seizures are generally believed to be induced by physical activity with the exception of one rare type of seizure disorder	

Key Points	*Subpoints*	*Examples*
	2. Whether or not an individual suffering from epilepsy should engage in a specific sport must be determined on an individual basis using common sense and advice from a sports medicine physician	
Sport conditioning for children	1. Children engaged in endurance sports respond in a manner comparable to that of adults, and there is no evidence to suggest that endurance training is harmful to children 2. Physical training has been shown to augment growth in children; however, how much physical training a child can engage in without harm to the musculoskeletal system remains controversial	
Women and training	1. Although many questions concerning the female athlete remain unanswered, there is little reason to limit the female from sports participation	
	2. The incidence of athletic amenorrhea appears to be highest in ballet dancers and distance runners	3% of the general female population experiences amenorrhea, whereas the incidence of amenorrhea in distance runners is 24%

Key Points	*Subpoints*	*Examples*
	3. A definitive answer to the cause of menstrual cycle dysfunction in athletes is not currently available. However, high levels of training stress have been linked to an increased incidence of athletic amenorrhea 4. Dysmenorrhea is believed to be due to prostaglandins. Athletes who experience mild dysmenorrhea can continue to train; however, athletes who experience severe dysmenorrhea should see a physician for treatment	
Training during pregnancy	1. Women who are physically fit prior to becoming pregnant can continue to perform mild or moderate (short-duration) exercise 2. Although controversial, at present, heavy exercise training is not recommended during pregnancy due to the possibility that intense exercise may reduce uterine blood flow	

Exam Questions

1. The key to safe participation in sports conditioning for the type I diabetic is to
   a. keep the intensity of the exercise low.
   b. perform only short-term high-intensity exercise.
   c. learn to avoid hypoglycemic episodes during training.
   d. learn to avoid small increases in blood glucose during training.

   c

2. Diabetic children do not respond to training in the same manner as do nondiabetic children.
   a. true
   b. false

   b

3. Children and adults with asthma can engage in physical conditioning and sports if they
   a. are able to control or prevent exercise-induced bronchospasms.
   b. train with other asthmatics.
   c. engage in low-intensity activities.
   d. None of the above are correct.

   a

4. At present, the recommendation for sports participation for epileptics is that
   a. the epileptic can participate in any sport when accompanied by a nonepileptic.
   b. individuals with only mild seizure problems and with the aid of proper medication can participate in most sports activities without harm.
   c. the individual should limit physical activity to low-intensity sports.
   d. epileptics should not participate in sports.

   b

5. Heavy endurance training in children has been shown to
   a. increase the risk of cardiovascular failure.
   b. decrease the risk of pulmonary disease.
   c. cause permanent musculoskeletal damage in 49% of the cases studied.
   d. None of the above are correct.

   d

6. It is generally believed that regular but not excessive physical activity in children promotes optimal bone growth and development.
   a. true
   b. false

   a

7. The occurrence of irregular menses in athletes is generally lower in swimmers when compared to
   a. cyclers.
   b. table tennis players.
   c. distance runners.
   d. None of the above are correct.

   c

8. It is generally agreed women can perform moderate-intensity (short-term) exercise during pregnancy.
   a. true
   b. false

   a

Chapter 23 Nutrition, Body Composition, and Performance

Lecture Outline

Key Points	*Subpoints*	*Examples*
Carbohydrate diets and performance	1. Supercompensation	Very high carbohydrate diet increases muscle glycogen store and extends performance
	2. Carbohydrates prior to performance	Take in 1 to 5 gm/kg to top off carbohydrate stores
	3. Carbohydrate ingestion during exercise	Extends performance by providing a higher rate of carbohydrate oxidation during exercise
Protein requirements exercise	1. Role of carbohydrate	Low carbohydrate stores increase the rate at which amino acids are used for energy
	2. Protein requirement for athletes	Higher than that of sedentary individuals; diet appears to be adequate
Water and electrolyte replacement during exercise	1. Ingest water before exercise	Top off body stores
	2. Ingest water/electrolyte drinks during exercise	Lowers heart rate and body temperature; recommended that drinks be cold; exercise less than 65%–70% $\dot{V}O_2$ max does not affect absorption
	3. Glucose content of drinks	Solutions of 10% or less are absorbed as fast as water during prolonged exercise

Key Points	*Subpoints*	*Examples*
Mineral needs with exercise	1. Salt needs in performance	Weigh in each day to make sure sodium needs are being met; if more sodium is needed; simply add salt to food at mealtimes
	2. Iron needs of athletes	It is difficult for a female athlete to maintain iron stores; analysis of blood would provide state of iron balance and supplementation may be needed
Vitamins and exercise	1. Is more needed?	If on a balanced diet, no supplementation is needed; if a true deficiency exists, then supplementation will help
	2. Toxicity	Large doses of fat soluble vitamins and vitamin C can cause problems
Pregame meal	1. Purpose	Top off water and carbohydrate stores, avoid hunger sensations, and prevent G.I. tract upset
	2. Composition	500–1000 kcal; very high in carbohydrate and low in protein and fat; can use prepared liquid meals
Somatotype and performance	1. Components	Endomorphy, mesomorphy, and ectomorphy
	2. Comparisons	Athletes are more mesomorphic than university students

Key Points	*Subpoints*	*Examples*
Body fatness and performance	1. Comparison with average person	Athletes tend to be leaner than their less athletically involved counterparts
	2. Norms	The average value listed for a group of athletes must be used as a guide since any team will have a range of values

Exam Questions

1. During heavy exercise lasting less than 2 hours, the primary fuel for muscular work is
   a. blood glucose.
   b. plasma FFA.
   c. muscle glycogen.
   d. amino acids.
   c

2. "Supercompensation" refers to the
   a. increase in muscle mass following heavy exercise.
   b. increase in muscle glycogen when exhaustive exercise is followed by a high-carbohydrate diet.
   c. procedures for paying subjects who are engaged in exhaustive exercise studies.
   d. consumption of a high-protein diet following weight training to increase muscle mass.
   b

3. The ingestion of carbohydrates during prolonged (2+ hours) increases time to exhaustion.
   a. true
   b. false
   a

4. The condition that has occurred in ultra-endurance (4+ hours) events when water, alone, is used to replace fluid loss is _____.
   hyponatremia

5. The normal daily protein requirement is
   a. $0.6 \text{ gm} \bullet \text{kg}^{-1}$.
   b. $0.8 \text{ gm} \bullet \text{kg}^{-1}$.
   c. $1.2 \text{ gm} \bullet \text{kg}^{-1}$.
   d. $1.6 \text{ gm} \bullet \text{kg}^{-1}$.
   b

6. Which of the following conditions increases the rate of amino acid utilization during exercise, as measured by an increased rate of nitrogen excretion in sweat?
   a. low-carbohydrate diet
   b. high-carbohydrate diet
   c. high-fat diet
   d. low-protein diet
   a

7. Since athletes need more protein than the average sedentary individual, athletes need to increase the amount of protein in their diets.
   a. true
   b. false
   b

8. Which of the following statements are true, relative to fluids taken during exercise? More than one answer may be true.
   a. Cold drinks are absorbed faster than warm drinks.
   b. Small volumes (about 200 ml) are absorbed faster than large volumes (about 600 ml).
   c. A glucose concentration of less than 10% does not interfere with the absorption of water.
   d. Exercise, independent of intensity, has no effect on the absorption of H_2O.

   a,c

9. Women athletes are more likely to have an iron deficiency because their dietary iron intake is inadequate.
   a. true
   b. false

   a

10. The vitamin that athletes need in an amount greater than the sedentary individual is
    a. vitamin A.
    b. niacin.
    c. riboflavin.
    d. None of the above are correct.

    d

11. Which of the following should not be included in the pregame meal?
    a. large amounts of protein
    b. large amounts of complex carbohydrates
    c. low amounts of fat

    a

12. The term associated with the linearity of one's body frame is
    a. ectomorphy.
    b. mesomorphy.
    c. endomorphy.

    a

13. When Olympic track and field athletes are compared to university students, the athletes tend to be located more in the
    a. mesomorphy area.
    b. ectomorphy area.
    c. endomorphy area.

    a

14. The optimum body fatness for male athletes is
    a. 8%.
    b. 10%.
    c. 12%.
    d. dependent on the sport and individual.

    d

Chapter 24 Exercise and the Environment

Lecture Outline

Key Points	*Subpoints*	*Examples*
Altitude affects performance	1. Changes in PO_2, air density, and temperature with altitude	All decrease with altitude
	2. Effect of altitude on sprint and endurance performance	Sprint performance may improve due to low air density; endurance performance decreases due to lower $\dot{V}O_2$ max
	3. Change in $\dot{V}O_2$ max with increasing altitude	Decrease in $\dot{V}O_2$ max is due to lower PO_2, which affects the saturation of hemoglobin; at higher altitudes, the lower maximal heart rate also influences response
	4. Effect of altitude on the heart rate and ventilation responses to submaximal exercise	Both are elevated at any given oxygen uptake at altitude
Adaptation to altitude	1. Adaptation to red blood cell production	Increases with altitude exposure
	2. Altitude natives vs. lowlanders who spend only a few years at altitude	Altitude natives show complete adaptation with $\dot{V}O_2$ max the same as those who live at sea level
	3. Variability in decrease in $\dot{V}O_2$ max in athletes who perform at altitude	May be due to the variability in the desaturation of hemoglobin; some athletes show this at sea level
	4. Athletes training at altitude	Detraining is possible due to reduced intensity and duration of training

Key Points	*Subpoints*	*Examples*
Climbing Mt. Everest without oxygen	$\dot{V}O_2$ max was higher than expected	Barometric pressure was higher than predicted, leading to higher PO_2 values and a higher $\dot{V}O_2$ max
Factors increasing heat injury	1. Environment, clothing, acclimatization, fitness, work load, and dehydration	Elevated temperatures and humidity, impermeable clothing, lack of water, and high work intensities increase risk; fit subjects tolerate heat better and acclimatize faster
	2. Running races on hot and humid days	Follow ACSM guidelines
	3. Heat stress index	Composed of wet bulb, globe, and dry bulb temperatures; wet bulb (an index of our ability to evaporate sweat) is most important
Factors related to hypothermia	1. Environment, clothing, and fitness	Low temperatures, wind, water, and a lack of fitness all contribute to hypothermia
	2. Windchill index	Effective temperature is lower than expected when wind is present due to increased heat loss by evaporation and convection
	3. Heat loss in cold air vs. cold water	Heat is lost about twenty-five times faster in cold water compared to air
	4. Clothing, body fatness, and energy production influence heat loss	Fat people lose heat slower than thin people; wearing clothing in layers minimizes sweating; lying down in the cold accelerates the decrease in body temperature

Key Points	*Subpoints*	*Examples*
Pollution and performance	Carbon monoxide	Binds to hemoglobin two hundred times more readily than O_2, decreasing the oxygen content of blood

Exam Questions

1. The PO_2 decreases with increasing altitude because of the
   a. lower percent of oxygen in the air.
   b. lower barometric pressure.
   c. Both (a) and (b) are correct.
   b

2. When track meets are held at altitude, the sprint performances are usually better than at sea level because of the
   a. lower PO_2.
   b. greater reliance on creatine phosphate for energy.
   c. greater reliance on anaerobic glycolysis for energy.
   d. lower air density.
   d

3. Distance-running performances are generally not as good when conducted at high altitude. This is due to the
   a. lower PO_2.
   b. greater reliance on creatine phosphate for energy.
   c. greater reliance on anaerobic glycolysis for energy.
   d. lower air density.
   a

4. Maximal aerobic power decreases with altitude due to the
   a. lower PO_2.
   b. lower percent of oxygen in the air.
   c. lower hemoglobin levels.
   d. increase in hemoglobin levels.
   a

5. Compared to the value measured at sea level, when a subject works at the same work rate at 3,000 meters altitude, the heart rate is
   a. higher
   b. lower.
   c. the same.
   d. dependent on the conditioning state of the subject.
   a

6. If maximal exercise is conducted at 21,000 feet altitude, $\dot{V}O_2$ max may be lower due to an actual reduction in maximal heart rate.
   a. true
   b. false
   a

7. Pulmonary ventilation is higher at altitude than at sea level for any work rate. This is necessary due to the
   a. colder air.
   b. lower air density.
   c. lower O_2 percentage.
   d. increased viscosity of the air.

   b

8. Natives that have resided at altitude all their lives adapt to the altitude by
   a. regular exercise.
   b. decreasing maximal ventilation.
   c. increasing the environmental PO_2.
   d. producing more red blood cells.

   d

9. Some athletes experience a larger than expected decrease in $\dot{V}O_2$ max when tested at altitude. This may be due to a
   a. larger desaturation of hemoglobin.
   b. greater decrease in maximal heart rate.
   c. greater decrease in maximal stroke volume.
   d. poor mitochondrial function.

   a

10. When Messner and Habeler climbed Mount Everest without supplemental oxygen, the scientists had to reevaluate their calculations that $\dot{V}O_2$ max at the top of Everest was equal to resting metabolic rate ($3.5 \text{ ml} \cdot \text{kg}^{-1} \cdot \text{min}^{-1}$). They found that the
    a. barometric pressure was higher than expected at the top of Everest.
    b. oxygen percentage was higher than expected at the top of Everest.
    c. the air temperature was colder than expected.
    d. the hemoglobin levels increased suddenly at that altitude for those who didn't use supplemental oxygen.

    a

11. Acclimatization to the heat results in an increased rate of sweating during exercise.
    a. true
    b. false

    a

12. When environmental temperature exceeds skin temperature,
    a. heat is gained by the body through convection and/or radiation.
    b. the sweat rate decreases.
    c. the sweat rate increases.
    d. Both (a) and (c) are correct.

    d

13. In the heat stress equation, which of the following terms are given the most consideration in predicting the heat load?
    a. dry bulb temperature
    b. black globe temperature
    c. wet bulb temperature

    c

14. The term that describes the potential loss of heat due to a combination cold air and air movement is
    a. hypothermia.
    b. frostbite.
    c. windchill.

    c

15. Which of the following individuals would lose heat faster when floating in cold water?
    a. thin athletic person
    b. fat sedentary person

    a

16. Carbon monoxide can decrease $\dot{V}O_2$ max by
    a. binding to hemoglobin to displace oxygen.
    b. irritating the bronchioles.
    c. decreasing the number of red blood cells.
    d. decreasing the arterial PO_2 to half its normal value.

    a

Chapter 25 Ergogenic Aids

Lecture Outline

Key Points	*Subpoints*	*Examples*
Definition of ergogenic aid	Work-producing	Blood doping
Research design concerns	1. Double-blind design	Neither subject nor investigator knows who received the substance
	2. Placebo	Use a "look-alike" substance or treatment to control for psychological factors
	3. Subject selection	Should be consistent with the purpose of the study, e.g., use elite runners rather than sedentary subjects
	4. Task	Use a task similar or identical to what the ergogenic aid is to influence
Supplemental oxygen and performance	1. Before exercise	O_2 breathing needs to take place two minutes prior to exercise, and effect is lost if breathing occurs
	2. During exercise	Performance is increased if oxygen is administered during exercise, possibly due to less H^+ formation
	3. After exercise	No evidence to support faster recovery with oxygen

Key Points	*Subpoints*	*Examples*
Blood doping and performance	1. Blood storage problems	"Old" technique could preserve blood for only three weeks, while the freezing method allows storage for years
	2. Achieving elevated hemoglobin concentrations	Subject needed time to naturally restore own blood prior to reinfusion; two units of blood were needed to see changes in $\dot{V}O_2$ max and performance
Blood buffers and performance	Buffering of lactic acid can improve performance in anaerobic events	Variability in improvements in performance; diarrhea and vomiting can occur
Amphetamines and performance	1. Physiological effects	Stimulate the central nervous system and act like catecholamines
	2. Mechanism of action	May spare muscle glycogen by mobilizing FFA; may mask the perception of fatigue
	3. Do they work?	Extends endurance and hastens recovery from fatigue; may be counterproductive in alert subjects by making them irritable
Caffeine and performance	1. Mechanism of action	Can directly stimulate skeletal muscle and the CNS and mobilize FFA to spare carbohydrate
	2. Ergogenic effect?	Dose dependent (7–15 mg/kg); pattern of use by the subject affects results; tests need to be field tests rather than laboratory tests to prove point

Key Points	*Subpoints*	*Examples*
Cocaine and its risks	1. Physiological effects	Powerful stimulator of the central nervous system and the cardiovascular system; very addictive
	2. Can cause psychological problems and death	Drug can cause paranoia, insomnia, and hallucinations and can lead to death via seizures and cardiac arrhythmias
Nicotine and performance	1. Physiological effects	Mixed effects due to the fact that the drug can activate both sympathetic and parasympathetic nervous systems
	2. Dangers	Addictive; if taken by smoking there is an increased risk of lung cancer and cardiovascular disease; if taken by chewing there is a risk of tooth decay, and gum disease, including cancers
Warm-up and performance	1. Types of warm-up	Indirect (general), direct (similar to task to be performed), and identical to task
	2. Mechanism of action	Higher body temperature facilitates enzyme action; increases arousal to optimum point
	3. Intensity and duration	For performance, the warm-up should be 60%–80% $\dot{V}O_2$ max for 10 minutes

Exam Questions

1. A double-blind research design is one in which
   a. the subject does not know which treatment he/she has been administered.
   b. both the subject and the investigator know what treatment had been administered.
   c. neither the subject nor the investigator know what treatment had been administered.
   d. only the investigator knows what treatment has been administered.

   c

2. Oxygen has been shown to be an effective ergogenic aid under the following circumstance:
   a. when the O_2 can be breathed during an endurance exercise.
   b. when O_2 is used before endurance exercise.
   c. when O_2 has been used in recovery from endurance exercise.

   a

3. Early studies did not show a positive effect of blood doping because
   a. too little blood was given to the subject.
   b. a significant portion of the red blood cells were destroyed during storage of the blood.
   c. the subject could not tolerate the additional blood.
   d. Both (a) and (b) are correct.

   d

4. The term *homologous transfusion* means that the subject received
   a. his own blood.
   b. a matched donor's blood.
   c. an artificial blood.

   b

5. How many units of blood had to be returned to the subject to show a positive effect of blood doping?
   a. .5 unit
   b. 1 unit
   c. 1.5 units
   d. 2 units

   d

6. Blood buffers, used to improve anaerobic performances, exert their effect by
   a. slowing the rate of decrease of creatine phosphate.
   b. slowing the rate of increase in plasma H^+.
   c. altering the rate at which oxygen leaves the hemoglobin.
   d. decreasing the rate at which H^+ leaves muscle.

   b

7. Amphetamines appear to have a positive effect on performance in those who are alert and motivated.
   a. true
   b. false

   b

8. The mechanism by which amphetamines may improve endurance performance is by
   a. increasing the use of plasma FFA.
   b. masking signs of fatigue.
   c. increasing arousal.
   d. All of the above are correct.

   d

9. Caffeine has been shown to have a variable effect on performance. This could be due to
   a. the amount of caffeine ingested.
   b. the subject's pattern of caffeine use.
   c. Both (a) and (b) are correct.

   c

10. The use of chewing tobacco to obtain a nicotine high may also be associated with which of the following problems?
    a. teeth and gum disease
    b. hair loss
    c. superficial twitching in the fingers and toes.
    d. Both (a) and (c) are correct.

    a

11. The recommended intensity of indirect warm-up for endurance activities is
    a. at 100% race pace.
    b. 60%–80% $\dot{V}O_2$ max.
    c. 40%—60% $\dot{V}O_2$ max.
    d. intervals exceeding race pace.

    b

12. When fire fighters warmed up prior to maximal exercise, there was
    a. a decrease in muscle soreness.
    b. an elimination of ST-segment depression.
    c. an increase in the number of ventricular beats.

    b